Contents

A Toss of the Dice

Stories from a Pediatrician's Practice

Natasha T. Hays

Jessica Kingsley Publishers
London and Philadelphia

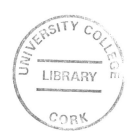

The author would like to thank the following publishers for permission to reproduce copyright material:
Viking Penguin, a division of Penguin Group (USA) Inc., and Penguin UK for the quotes on page 11 from *The Cunning Man* by Robertson Davies, copyright © 1994 Robertson Davies, and on page 144 from *What's Bred in the Bone* by Robertson Davies, copyright © 1985 Robertson Davies.
Viking Penguin, a division of Penguin Group (USA) Inc., and the author for the quote on page 75 from *Ordinary People* by Judith Guest, copyright © 1976 Judith Guest.
Hap-Pal Music for the quote on page 85 from the CD "Peek-A-Boo" and video "Baby Songs" by Hap Palmer and Martha Cheney © 1983 Hap-Pal Music. Available at www.happalmer.com
Random House, Inc., and Time Warner Book Group UK for the quote on page 130–1 from *I Know Why the Caged Bird Sings* by Maya Angelou, copyright © 1969 and renewed 1997 Maya Angelou.
Houghton Mifflin Company and IMG-BACH for the quote on page 136 from *The Prince of Tides* by Pat Conroy, copyright © 1986 Pat Conroy. All rights reserved.

The right of Natasha T. Hays to be identified as author of this work has been asserted by her in accordance with the Copyright, Designs and Patents Act 1988.

First published in 2003 by 1stBooks

This edition first published in 2005
by Jessica Kingsley Publishers
116 Pentonville Road
London N1 9JB, UK
and
400 Market Street, Suite 400
Philadelphia, PA 19106, USA

www.jkp.com

Copyright © Natasha T. Hays 2005

Library of Congress Cataloging in Publication Data

Hays, Natasha T. (Natasha Thomasovna), 1956–
 A toss of the dice : stories from a pediatrician's practice / Natasha T. Hays.-- Rev. ed.
 p. ; cm.
 Includes bibliographical references and index.
 ISBN 1-84310-788-0 (pbk.)
 1. Pediatrics--Anecdotes. 2. Developmentally disabled children--Anecdotes.
 [DNLM: 1. Pediatrics--Personal Narratives. WZ 100 H425t 2005] I. Title.
 RJ47.H44 2005
 618.92--dc22

                                                            2004011538

British Library Cataloguing in Publication Data
A CIP catalogue record for this book is available from the British Library

ISBN-13: 978 1 84310 788 0
ISBN-10: 1 84310 788 0

Printed and Bound in Great Britain by
Athenaeum Press, Gateshead, Tyne and Wear

Acknowledgements

Many thanks to my sister, Kim Hays, who read through my manuscript with an editor's eye and made invaluable suggestions. She is finally forgiven for breaking my toy parachute. I also thank my parents, Joy and Tom Hays, and my uncle, Kimball Kramer, for adding their helpful two cents' worth here and there.

My husband, Phil Whitworth, remained supportive and encouraging throughout the project and was invaluable in helping me with computer glitches. I also thank my children, Ariel and Alex, for allowing me to put in anecdotes about their childhood. I appreciate all that they taught me about being a good mother and pediatrician. They are turning out to be adults that I would choose for my friends.

I wish to thank the dedicated and compassionate colleagues who have worked with me at the Developmental Evaluation Centers in Morganton, Hickory, and Shelby.

And lastly, I thank the children who have been my patients. They have given me more than I could ever give them. I hope that my doctoring has added to their lives in some way.

The patients in this book are mainly composite characters taken from several different patients with similar problems. In all cases, names and details have been changed to protect confidentiality.

Chapter 1

News by Telephone

It was the kind of phone call that made you feel as if someone had just punched you in the stomach.

I had been dreaming. It had been a particularly difficult day, with several children with behavior problems whom I had had to chase around to do their physicals. There had also been a hostile father who came to the office to tell me that his wife was telling me lies about him. I was home from work and taking a much-needed nap. All these events were somehow caught up in my dream and the ringing of the phone took a little while to penetrate my brain. Still groggy, I picked up the phone. I could feel my heart pounding from being so suddenly awakened.

"Hello, Dr. Hays?" said a familiar voice. "This is Janice Guffey. I'm not calling about Anthony this time. It's Caitlin. I don't know – it's just that something's not right about the way she moves. When can you see her?"

The Guffeys were an attractive couple in their early thirties. Jake Guffey worked as a plant manager and Janice had been a schoolteacher until they had their first child, Anthony. It was an easy pregnancy and a perfect, full-term delivery. They were adoring parents and did everything the books said to do and more to help Anthony thrive.

It had come as a terrible shock when, at about eight months, they realized that Anthony was not sitting up or babbling as he should have been doing about two months before and, also, that he had begun to shake and bob when he tried to move. His eyes also danced back and forth in a crazy rhythm.

They took him to their pediatrician. Not knowing what was wrong, but looking for a place to start, she referred him to us, the Developmental Evaluation Center (DEC).

The couple were waiting anxiously in the waiting room when we ushered them into the comfortable area we use for parent conferences.

"What's wrong with our baby?" Mrs. Guffey asked. "Can you tell us what's going on?"

I leaned forward and tried to steel myself to being the bearer of bad news, by far the hardest part of my job.

"Anthony has 'ataxia.' This means that the balance and coordination areas of the brain are damaged and are causing him to have trouble with balance and changes in position. It is also what is causing the overall body trembling and trouble reaching."

"What can we do about it?" asked Mr. Guffey, putting a comforting hand over his wife's.

"We know what he has and we can give him physical therapy to help him to cope with his difficulty with balance, but we don't, at this point, know what is causing the ataxia. That's what we need to find out. It may be something treatable and we need to know that as soon as possible so that we can be sure that it doesn't get any worse."

"Did I do something wrong while I was pregnant? I don't think I was sick at all and it was an easy birth. He did great."

"It may be that there was some sort of difficulty during your pregnancy, but this seems to have started when he was about six months. Before that he wasn't having any problems. That would not be typical for a child who had some sort of problem before or during the birth process."

"There's something else. I'm not sure how well Anthony can see and I want to check that out with a specialist."

The Guffeys wanted to do everything possible to test Anthony to determine a diagnosis.

We sent him to an ophthalmologist, who confirmed what we had suspected. Anthony was what is called "cortically blind," which means that there is nothing wrong with the eyes but that the part of the brain that interprets shapes and colors and turns them into meaningful information is not working well.

Then began the doctor shuffle. What was going on with Anthony's brain? It might be some sort of metabolic disorder. It might be genetic. Did the Guffeys have anybody on either side of the family who had shown similar symptoms? No, they weren't aware of anyone. Anyone who had experienced stillbirths or miscarriages? Again, no. Were they related? No, except in the way that everyone in McDowell County was related way back. Guffey was a very common name.

Anthony went from neurologist to geneticist and then to another neurologist and another geneticist at a bigger hospital, and finally did one more round at a famous medical center. Many tests were done but no one found any more specific diagnosis or cause of Anthony's symptoms. All anyone could tell them was that Anthony had ataxia. Finally, the Guffeys said enough was enough. If this was something that no one knew how to treat, why should they continue to make poor Anthony suffer? They would give him physical therapy and get him services for the blind and do everything else to help him and make his life happy, but that was it.

One thing they heard from the genetic counselor was that, as far as he knew, there was no reason to think that if they were to have another child he or she would have similar problems. Or at least, that is what the Guffeys heard him say. I was not there, so I can't know what was said. So they had Caitlin.

I am always glad when a family who has a child with special needs has another child who is developmentally normal. It is delightful for them to see the second child grow and develop as expected but, even more importantly, it often takes pressure off them and also off their disabled child to achieve at an expected level. It helps them to appreciate both children more. They realize that they are not to blame for the child's disabilities and they can enjoy his personality and personal progress.

Caitlin was also a beautiful baby, with big brown eyes and her mother's curly red hair. Anthony loved to stroke her hair and to feel her face. She laughed and smiled early. At Christmas, they sent us a picture of the children, Anthony with his hand on Caitlin's shoulder, staring into space, but smiling, and Caitlin propped up on the photographer's pillows, wearing a red velvet dress with a lace collar.

Then, when Caitlin was 13 months, that anxious call from Mrs. Guffey came.

The physical therapist, Lela, and I saw Caitlin at once. Yes, it was clear that she was having some problems. She sat and crawled, but she seemed very hesitant to move and she, too, had a tendency to bob and sway. We gently told them that we wanted them to see a neurologist, but that we did feel it was very likely that she had the same problem that Anthony had and that it must be hereditary, probably an autosomal recessive condition, each parent contributing a faulty gene, since it had never occurred in either family before.

The Guffeys were understandably overwhelmed. Our hopes and dreams for our children are deeply felt by all parents. When we realize our children cannot fully achieve what we had hoped for them, it is a grief that tears at our hearts. When two children in the family have disabilities, the grief is more than doubled. Fortunately they had a lot of family and community support and were able to work through their grief and come to an acceptance about their tragedy. They are a very loving family and have been able to get the best of services for both Anthony and Caitlin. They have had no further children. Both children are a pleasure, affectionate and happy, with beautiful manners and good social skills, and we always enjoy seeing them when they come for exams or physical therapy. Still, it was hard for them to understand why this had happened to them. It was hard for me, too – and still is.

I have also seen the exact opposite situation, a family who has been warned not to have other children and who went on to have two or three normally developing boys and girls. The bottom line is that having children is just a toss of the dice. We all carry quite a few seeds for genetic disorders in our chromosomes. It depends on the combination of those chromosomes and those of our mate and we can only hope for the best. "There but for the grace of God, go I" was never a more apt saying than in this situation.

Working with people like the Guffeys has taught me of the strength and courage that families can find when faced with a tragedy of this magnitude. They usually manage to get beyond their grief about not having the "perfect child" that they had dreamed about and are able simply to enjoy the child they have. And my colleagues and I, in working with special needs children day in and day out, have learned what a delight they can be and how rewarding it is to help them live up to their potential.

Chapter 2

Medical School

I believe, as I discovered Paracelsus had believed before me, that there are as many stomachs, hearts, livers, and lights as there are members of the human race, and that they should be treated individually to suit their special needs, whatever these might be. Treatment must be intensely personal, and if sometimes it strays into the realm of mind, there the physician must follow it.

Robertson Davies, The Cunning Man

My own childhood doctor, Dr. Cuevas, was an exceptionally sweet Puerto Rican man who was a family practitioner. I always enjoyed going to see him. I'd get a warm embrace from him and he'd always say,

"And how is my Natasha today?"

He showed a humorous understanding of the effect of environment on health and mental health. Both my sister Kim and I bit our nails as children. My mother tried everything to get us to stop from putting pepper on our fingertips to offering bribes. And of course she nagged. Finally she went to Dr. Cuevas to ask for his advice.

He paused and looked at my mother, all five feet of her bristling with energy and high expectations, her long list of things to do that day in her hand.

"Joy," he said, shaking his head. "Leave them alone. If I had to live with you and Tom, I'd bite my nails, too."

She took the hint. Kim and I were forever grateful to him, and I don't bite my nails anymore.

I had warm relationships with other doctors in my life, too, but it had not occurred to me to become a doctor, there being no health professionals of any sort in my family and, in fact, four Christian Science grandparents who did not believe in doctors at all.

It was not until my junior year at Oberlin College, Ohio, that I decided that I wanted to be a doctor instead of doing psychobiological research, which was what I had originally planned. Although I enjoyed it, research had its problems for me. I was a person who enjoyed being active and working directly with people. I had always found that I was good at listening to people's troubles and that, in fact, people sought me out to talk. It came to me that I was far more suited to being a physician.

I began medical school in 1977 at the University of North Carolina, Chapel Hill, and finished at the University of Minnesota because my husband, Phil, began his internship there, and I followed. I feel I had the best of both worlds because the professors at Chapel Hill were fascinating and the University of Minnesota was a medical Mecca that brought patients from all over the United States.

The first two years of medical school involve an enormous amount of studying, as well as the initiation into the scientific understanding of the human body. This begins with the dissection of a cadaver. I remember the solemn, slightly frightened feeling (and the formaldehyde preservative) that permeated the air as we approached the room we would be spending half our lives in for the first year. This experience may harden some students, but it also creates awe at the complex make-up of a human being. We also had classes on every aspect of medicine. The study of the brain was particularly interesting to me, because it was that small organ that made everything else function. The brain had so many jobs and there were so many ways that something could go wrong and change a person's life forever. Now I see examples of that every day.

When you start clinical rotations in medical school, you find yourself drawn to certain areas of medicine. A lot of it has to do with how interesting the professors (or attending physicians) are, but even more of it has to do with your personality. Certain types of people tend to gravitate to particular fields. Orthopedists are usually muscular people interested in sports. Obstetricians particularly like women and babies. Psychiatrists are more interested in the humanities in many cases and look at medical school as a means to an end. Internists are usually interested in details and in putting together pieces of information. Emergency Room (ER) doctors and surgeons tend to like the adrenaline rush that comes with saving a life in a crisis situation. Obviously these are stereotypes, but there's something to them all.

I did not think much of surgery. There was a very rigid hierarchy of authority and the medical student was way at the bottom. Students were left to hold incisions open with retractors and were lucky if they were allowed to look some of the time at what was going on. I did get to put in enormous numbers of intravenous (IV) lines. Doctors and nurses in training will identify with the experience of looking at people's veins at a party, on the bus, while eating lunch, anywhere, and thinking, "He has good veins. They'd be easy to stick" or "Wow! I sure wouldn't want to try getting an IV into that guy."

Internal medicine was very interesting and I had excellent teaching, but it didn't quite seem like me. It was too serious. Radiology was more relaxing; however, I missed the patient interaction.

I certainly enjoyed helping with deliveries. The excitement of a new baby coming into the world is never stale. I also had very nice residents on obstetrics and gynecology who taught me a lot and were patient. I could see myself doing that, but gynecology had a lot more routine-type work, and waiting for a mother to begin delivering could be a very long and unpredictable process.

Best of all, I found, I liked the pediatricians and the child psychiatrists. The pediatricians seemed like gentle folks with good senses of humor and an ability to express their feelings. The child psychiatrists were similar, but with a more philosophic view of life and drier sense of humor. While on my child psychiatry rotation I was taking care of a child on the ward who was felt to have "hysterical cerebral palsy" and who was showing great difficulty walking and talking. I happened to fall down the stairs and sprain my ankle during that rotation. As I came hobbling in on crutches the next day, my attending physician looked at me wryly.

"Can you still talk?" he asked.

What is fascinating and also very sad about that case is that now, knowing more about pediatric neurology, I am convinced that the little girl had a disease called "muscularum deformans," and not a disorder that was "all in her head." I hope she did all right. There are patients that continue to haunt you well after you have lost track of them because you feel you failed them in some way.

On my pediatric rotation I met several physicians at Minneapolis Children's Hospital who were people I wanted to emulate. I once watched one of them, Dr. Dan Kohen, interview a child who had been sexually abused and, in his careful and quiet way, pull information out of her that she had never told anyone else. It was he who taught me that the interview is by far the most important and essential part of reaching a diagnostic conclusion.

I also did a rotation in pediatrics at Saint Paul Ramsey, a county hospital. Here we generally saw poorer patients from many ethnic groups. My Puerto Rican Spanish and high-school French came in handy. I also still remember my one word of Hmong: "Chu!" which means "push!" – useful for deliveries! The women in labor brought their women relatives with them, and we doctors just waited on the sidelines to make sure that the baby was all right.

Another mentor, Dr. Tom Rolewicz, was in charge of the head trauma unit at Ramsey, among other things. With him, we saw children who had been thrown from cars or fallen out of trees and who often remained in a coma for weeks. After the urgency of emergency treatment to keep the pressure from building up too seriously in the brain, there was the long wait for them to wake up, bit by bit. Then the even longer rehabilitation to bring them back to their previous state of running, laughing, talking, and remembering their school lessons. Sometimes a child suddenly woke up and was fine, almost as if he or she had awakened from a nap. Usually not.

One lesson we were all taught on that rotation was that people in coma may be more awake than you know. Though they may not be able to respond to anything in their environment, they may hear everything that is said.

One child who woke from a coma remembered that a resident had come in and said, "This child isn't going to make it." He also remembered the nurse who stroked his hand throughout much of her shift and told him stories. He could repeat some of the stories.

Even more eerily, some of the children reported being able to hear and see things during the time that they were being resuscitated in the Emergency Room. The accuracy of their statements about what had been said and what had happened was enough to make anyone realize the brain and the soul are very mysterious things that we don't even begin fully to under-stand.

I learned to say to a child in a coma, "Hi Charlie. It's Dr. Hays again. Remember me? I was in here yesterday. Dr. Jones is here, too."

"How you doing, Charlie?"

"I'm going to check your pupils and listen to your heart now. It won't hurt."

I'd touch the child gently. "Can you hear me? If you can, try to squeeze my hand."

It was a moment of joy and relief when that feeble hand-squeeze occurred and another moment of celebration when their eyes opened.

What I found was that, on the pediatric ward, I enjoyed the children I got to spend time with. Children are always lovable, always beautiful, always changeable. They have incredible powers of recovery. They have an enormous capacity to learn and we learn important lessons from them, too. They are a pleasure to be with.

Chapter 3

Pediatric Residency

Grasp the slivery butterfly spear
Fix tube to syringe.
Deft, mustn't fumble.
Her tiny arm trembles, and slowly, one tear
Slides down that soft cheek.
We all watch it tumble,
Wetting the sheet.
Now feel for a vein:
That thin curling line, that fragile red river
Gives way to my fingers.
More tears, spreading stain.
("No Mommy, no!")
Her parents both shiver
As, quick, I pierce skin.
We inhale; red drop
Flows into my tube.
("Don't stick me! Oh stop!
Please make me get better, please promise!")
Blood spurts.
I can't promise, sweetheart.
It hurts. Please. It hurts.

Written during the author's residency

I decided that pediatrics was the place I belonged. The residency that was offered at the University of Minnesota was particularly diverse since the residents had the opportunity to work at five different types of hospitals. They ranged from the big university hospital that had very, very ill children with rare diseases where many experimental treatments were tried, to a county hospital that saw mainly poor people, to a city hospital that was run through private pediatricians. We also worked with private pediatricians in an office setting.

Most people have heard that being a medical intern and resident is incredibly difficult, and they are absolutely right. It is true that you don't get much sleep; you have enormous responsibilities for patients and are continually trying to keep up with learning so that you can do a good job. You don't see much of your family. You do end up crying in the hospital bathroom a lot because someone you cared about died, or you got yelled at, or you feel you goofed up, or you are just incredibly tired, or all of these at once.

I heartily approve of some of the changes that have been made in residency programs that limit the amount of time a resident has to be awake and still taking care of patients because it is more humane and, more importantly, fewer mistakes are made.

When I was an intern, we took care of a 13-year-old girl, Angie, with diabetes who had developed antibodies against her injected insulin and it seemed that no matter how much we gave her, her blood sugar wouldn't come down. She felt horrible and we felt helpless.

I called up my resident to tell him that her blood sugar was 425. He was in charge of all the pediatric wards at night and had probably had his beeper going off every ten minutes, running from one child to another, putting out fires, so to speak.

"Angie's blood sugar is 425 – I don't know what to do," I told him.

In a few minutes, he was down on the ward with his rumpled scrub suit and five o'clock shadow.

"What have you been doing?" he yelled at me. "Don't you know how to handle a blood sugar? You're never going to be a doctor if you don't start taking care of things. Do I have to babysit you all the time?"

After a stammered apology, I stumbled off to the call room with tears blurring my eyes. I vowed that when I was a resident, I wouldn't yell at my medical students and interns, no matter how stressed I was. I don't think I ever did either, though I was sorely tempted at times.

I remember comforting a medical student a few years later after a child she had been taking care of died. The mother had brought the child into the Emergency Room three times and she had been examined, treated, and sent out again. She just didn't look as sick as she truly was. The last time, the child was limp and unresponsive.

"The mother was right there, watching while we tried to bring her back," the student sobbed. "Every time her heartbeat would come back, she would cry out, 'Go, go!' and stare right at that monitor as her baby's heartbeat disappeared again."

"Everyone kept trying and trying to get her back and it kept not working and finally they just gave up. No one else cried," she said. "I feel like I'm so weak, but I just don't know if I can stand it. Does this mean that I'm not going to make it?"

"Hey," I told her. "We've all been there. We all cry sometimes. It shows that you have compassion for the children and the families."

"Even the guys cry sometime?" she asked.

"Even the guys. They just hide it more. Of course, some of them don't. But do you really want to harden yourself to the point that you don't care?"

"No," she said. "I guess I don't."

My husband, Phil, also learned a good bit of "medicine in the trenches" during his medical school years. He had several experiences that taught him that there is more than one way to do things and not to be too sure that your way is the right one in all cases.

Phil did his acting internship training towards the tail end of medical school in Franklin, a small town in western North Carolina with stunning mountain views and a gem-mining industry. He worked with an elderly country doctor who had probably seen every emergency situation known, and often had dealt with them in some primitive conditions.

One night, when Phil was taking the internist's place, he was called to the hospital for a cardiac arrest. He had never been in charge of an arrest before, but he had determined in his mind exactly what he would do in that situation.

He ran in.

"Let's give him…" and he reeled off his carefully memorized plan.

"But Doctor Johnson usually does this," said the nurse, giving him different orders.

"Well, let's do that then," he readily agreed. One can't be too humble in a learning situation!

Not only do you learn an enormous amount of medicine in residency, but also you learn an equal amount about listening to patients. You learn how to talk about very difficult topics.

One evening a family was sent down from the Northern Minnesota Iron Range to the "big city hospital" because of their baby's severe anemia. They had been told little else. When I examined the eight-month-old, I felt numb. His belly was protruding and his liver and spleen were huge. He was extremely pale, and he had what appeared to be two large shiners or "raccoon eyes." I was pretty sure he had cancer and furthermore, I was pretty sure it was neuroblastoma, which is very serious.

I sat down with the family, my medical students beside me, and I gently explained to them what I suspected and what we would be doing. They were stunned and we gave them time to cry and talk and ask questions. Still, after anyone hears very bad news there is a period of shock when you can't really think and don't always hear what else is said.

When we left the room, my medical students told me they thought I had handled the discussion very well. The attending physician came in the morning and, among other things, a bone-marrow biopsy and nuclear scan were planned.

It turned out that, indeed, the boy did have neuroblastoma, but he had "Stage IV-S",[1] which sometimes spontaneously goes away. At that time, it was not even always treated with chemotherapy, just with steroids. I was very relieved and rushed in to tell the good news to the parents.

"It's good news!" I said. "Marcus does have neuroblastoma, but he has the kind that often goes away on its own!"

The mother stared at me and burst into tears.

"My baby has cancer," she said, "and you think it's good news?"

Although the baby did get better, I feel sure that the mother never trusted me again. Good news to me was not good news to her, and in my relief that the diagnosis wasn't worse I had forgotten that. One can never be too careful about giving information in a sensitive manner.

Another misunderstanding – far more amusing – happened when I was working in the Neonatal Intensive Care Unit. A 15-year-old African-American girl had a baby quite prematurely, about two-and-a-half months early. Her mother, the grandmother of the baby, was only 30. Family history was repeating itself, and the grandmother, knowing what her daughter was giving up, was not too happy about it. Fortunately, the daughter's boyfriend had been there during the delivery and seemed to be an involved father.

The baby was on a ventilator but was doing very well and was expected to continue to improve with minimal complications. As I was finishing up my notes on the tiny little girl, the grandmother came up, tight-lipped and clearly very upset.

"What's wrong with the baby's color?" she asked.

I looked over and saw a baby with no blue tinge or dusky purplish color, two signs that would indicate that the baby was not getting enough oxygen.

"Absolutely nothing's wrong with the baby's color," I assured her. "She's doing fine."

The grandmother shook her head vigorously. She repeated, "What is wrong with the baby's color?"

I looked again and saw a beautifully pink baby with dark blue eyes. Suddenly, it occurred to me what she meant. She thought her daughter had been fooling around with a white boy!

"Oh!" I said. "Very premature babies haven't developed their pigment yet. There is nothing at all wrong. The baby is going to be getting darker – just you wait and see."

Sure enough the little girl darkened as she grew and by the time she left the hospital, she was close to the same skin color as her mother and grandmother. I was glad that I had saved the teenager from being flayed alive by her mother. Not everyone looks at a baby and sees what a doctor would consider important.

Chapter 4

More Lessons, Including Humility

On such a night, or such a night,
Would anybody care
If such a little figure
Slipped quiet from its chair.

So quiet, oh, how quiet!
That nobody might know
But that the little figure
Rocked softer, to and fro?

On such a dawn, or such a dawn,
Would anybody sigh
That such a little figure
Too sound asleep did lie?

Emily Dickinson, "On such a night, or such a night"

When a doctor works with a patient, especially a child, he or she is actually treating the whole family. The child has the disease, but it is the parents who deal with the anxiety of the illness and the difficult decisions to be made about their child. It is they with whom the doctor has to communicate most. However, I have always had the conviction that the child's health and safety come first. That is always my primary responsibility.

I was soon to discover how difficult that conflict could be. A lawyer and his wife, both fairly prominent in their community, rushed in their 11-month-old daughter, who was unconscious.

"Tara is just learning to walk," Mr. Andresen, the father, said, in a panic. "I was at home and my wife was at the store. I heard her crying. I ran to find her and she had fallen down the stairs. She had a cut on her nose, so I put a Bandaid on it. Then she calmed down, so I put her down for her nap."

"When I got home and went to check on her, she wasn't breathing!" Mrs. Andresen sobbed. "The paramedics got her breathing again when they came, but she hasn't opened her eyes and she doesn't know me. Is she going to be all right?"

The Emergency Room staff was madly putting in IVs and bagging the child with oxygen, the head ER doc barking out orders as fast as he could. They had to intubate her, put a tube down her windpipe in order for a ventilator to artificially breathe for her. Very soon she was in the Pediatric Intensive Care Unit (PICU) covered with tubes and tape and the other paraphernalia of the very ill child. Her skin was scraped and bruised from her stair fall. Even in her condition, she was a pretty little girl, with dark hair, dark eyes, and light brown skin. The parents were both typical Minnesotans, blond-haired and blue-eyed.

We removed the large Bandaid over her nose. That was the first clue that something was very, very wrong with the history of the injury. The "cut" on her nose was an enormous gash that practically cut her nose in two. No parent in his right mind would have just put a Bandaid on it and put her down for her nap. We alerted the Department of Social Services.

Tara lasted for four days before she died of massive swelling of the brain from traumatic brain injury with a resulting skull fracture and internal bleeding. During the time she was in the PICU right around Christmas, some of the Minnesota Vikings came to the wards to distribute stuffed animals to all the children. Although well meant, this was not a good idea on the PICU, where most of the children were critically ill or dying and would never need a toy again. It was very hard on all the parents. Tara was given a stuffed rabbit with floppy ears, which sat alone on a table in her room. She never had a chance to play with it.

The real story eventually came out. Tara was adopted from India at nine months. It was the mother who badly wanted a child and talked the father into adopting, since they could not have children of their own. The father often worked late, and when he came home he wanted to do his paperwork and relax. He found the baby's presence very irritating. He had even said something to me in the hospital about how "sometimes babies cry and cry and you just want to…" He didn't finish the sentence.

Then, a month after they brought Tara home, Mrs. Andresen discovered that she was pregnant. Mr. Andresen became still more resentful of the adopted baby and increasingly agitated when she cried.

He had confessed to his wife later that, when she went to the store, Tara wouldn't stop crying. In a moment of pure rage, he picked her up and threw her down the stairs. Then he was incredibly frightened at what he had done. He covered the bleeding gash and put her to bed, hoping against hope that things would be okay if he just pretended they hadn't happened. Mrs. Andresen was torn about whether she should protect her husband or not, but she eventually told Social Services what had happened.

As the attending physician testified in court, "Parents do abuse their children in stress and anger, even when they love them. But when they see what they have done, they rush their children to the Emergency Room. This father didn't even try to help her until her mother discovered Tara not breathing. This is murder."

I also had to testify to several of the unusual statements the father had made during the hospitalization and about Tara's condition when we first saw her. For some reason, the father's lawyer asked me for my address. I saw the father write it down, and then he gave me a slit-eyed look of hatred. I have never been so glad to see someone go to prison in my life.

Mrs. Andresen gave me the stuffed rabbit in remembrance of Tara. I still have it and I will never forget her or the lesson she taught me. Always be "sympathetically suspicious." Things are not always the way they look, and no socioeconomic class is exempt from child abuse.

During my residency I also learned about the bravery and maturity that extremely ill children could develop from their experiences. Jeffrey was a seven-year-old with a severe type of blood cancer, acute myelocytic leukemia, which, at that time, was very close to incurable if there was a relapse after the first remission.

Jeffrey's parents loved him a great deal and losing him was unthinkable. They were always at the hospital with him, they read to him, they suffered with him through his treatments. Eventually the doctors offered them the last option, a bone-marrow transplant. Bone-marrow transplantation was still in its infancy and the University of Minnesota was one of the few places where it was done. There were many risks, including overwhelming infection, bleeding, and the dreaded "graft-versus-host" disease, where the bone marrow itself begins attacking the "foreign" person's organs. The likelihood that he would be cured was much smaller than the likelihood that he would die.

Still, Jeffrey's parents wanted any possible chance for him to live and they agreed to the transplantation. Jeffrey was of a different mind.

"I've talked to other children on the station," he said. "I've seen children die. I've seen how sick they got before they died. I'm not scared of dying. I'm tired of hurting. I don't want to have the transplant."

Jeffrey's parents were torn when they heard his feelings, but they still chose for him to have the bone-marrow transplant. Jeffrey was calm about it, but he still maintained that he didn't want to go through with this. Seven-year-old children aren't supposed to have such a thoughtful attitude toward death, but this one did. He had a full appreciation of life, too.

At the time, I disagreed with his parents' choice. Now that I have children, I'm not by any means as positive. I probably would have done the same thing that they did. I do know that when my daughter Ariel was in the ICU with a severe disease that swells the throat and closes off the airway, called epiglottitis, I would have done anything, no matter how drastic, if someone told me it was the only chance to keep her alive. Thanks to intubation with tubes to keep her windpipe open, and antibiotics to fight the bacterial infection, she pulled through with no ill effects. She was very fortunate.

Jeffrey did not have her luck. On his last day, he turned to his mother and said, "Mama, I just want to go home. Can I go home?" She held his hand and quietly nodded. He smiled, squeezed her hand, and closed his eyes. He had died peacefully.

Minneapolis/St. Paul has the largest urban Native American population in the United States. Many of our patients, especially in the county hospitals, were Native Americans, and a number of them were still very involved in their indigenous culture and traditions. It was not unusual to be working with a child right along with the medicine man that the parents had asked be brought in. We were respectful of them and they of us.

One of the things that the medicine men did was to place an eagle feather at the top of the bed. If the feather curled up and shriveled this meant the child would die. If it stayed straight then the child would live. I later heard that a medicine man would wet the feather on one side if he felt it should curl up and the heat in the hospital did the rest. They had long experience with people who were ill and had a pretty good idea of who would live and who would die. This was their way of preparing a family. They were usually right.

I also knew several long-time ER nurses who were usually right. They were essentially trained doctors from their multiple experiences with patients. One woman who had worked for years and years as the head nurse and triage person at Minneapolis Children's Hospital, Rosie, was the best diagnostician I've ever come across.

"The patient with pneumonia's in Room 2," she'd say. "The one with pinworms is in Room 3. Is it okay if I have them start an IV on the child with meningitis in Room 6? You need to see him first."

All she had done was hear the initial history and look at the child and she knew what was wrong. We doctors listened to Rosie. She knew what she was talking about.

I remember one time in the ER when we were having an extra dose of chaos. I was taking care of a child who was having a febrile seizure when a father came in, carrying his small child in his arms. The child was beginning to shake and roll its eyes back and he was panicking. He began sobbing and yelling frantically for help.

"My son! Somebody take care of my son! Do something!"

Rosie stepped right in.

"Seizures when small children have a fever are common," she told him calmly. "I know they're scary, but they're common."

"See?" she said, leading him to the room where the other child was just getting over the febrile seizure and becoming quiet. "Look – lots of kids are having seizures here."

It was a technique I'd never thought of before, but it worked. The father became quieter, looked down at his son, and noted that the child was quietly asleep in his arms, a light sweat breaking out on his forehead. He would be okay.

Another evening a ten-year-old boy was hurriedly brought in by his parents. In evening dress and with their opera glasses around their necks, they had obviously come straight from the opera.

"Our older daughter called," the mother told us. "She told us that Jake said he had a bad stomach-ache and went to go to the bathroom. He called her to come and there was a whole toiletful of blood. They were both scared to death."

"Why is he bleeding from his bottom?" asked his father, worriedly.

Jake, in the meantime, appeared in no obvious physical distress but he was very frightened, perhaps even more by the worried adult faces than by his bloody diarrhea.

We hurried them into a room. If Jake had lost that much blood from his rectum, something must be very wrong.

There was a good bit of bloodstain on Jake's pajama pants and soon there was some on the pad covering the cot. Jake saw it and started to cry. I was also worried. The blood was bright red, which suggested that it was new and that he was bleeding rapidly.

"Am I going to bleed to death?" he sobbed.

Rosie looked at the blood. She wrinkled her forehead.

"Wait a minute," she said. She went to get a guaiac stain card that can detect small amounts of blood in stool. She tested the bloody stool on the pad. The guaiac card showed no evidence of blood.

"It looks too red," she said. "What did you have for dinner?"

"Well, Mom and Dad were out," he said, sniffling. "Lisa gave me cherry jello. She said it was okay!"

"How much cherry jello did you eat?" asked his mother.

"A big bowl."

"How big a bowl?"

"The – uh – the whole package," he said.

"It looks like you're having plain, ordinary diarrhea and that the jello ran right through you," I said, relieved that we weren't going to have to get the IVs going, call the surgeons, and begin typing blood for Jake.

"We left the opera for this?" his father asked, half laughing and half indignant. He playfully cuffed his son. "No more red jello for you!"

"I thought it looked too red," said Rosie, nodding.

Virtually any child who was hospitalized at our primary training center, the University of Minnesota Hospital, was guaranteed to be very sick, with cancer, severe diabetes, kidney failure, heart disease, cystic fibrosis, you name it. In fact, we had some children who had several diseases at once. I took care of a girl who had Down syndrome with Tetralogy of Fallot (an associated congenital heart disease) who also had cystic fibrosis. A lot of the children had been there so often for "tune-ups" that they knew all the staff and many of the other children and sort of considered the hospital a second home.

This was especially true of the children who had cystic fibrosis. It was interesting to see how they coped with their chronic illnesses, especially their body images. One teenager used to put on elaborate make-up every morning, curl her hair, and dress beautifully, even if she would just be lying in bed. Another boy lifted weights and had pictures of weightlifters in his room. This wouldn't be so unusual, but he was only nine years old.

A boy who had leukemia would allow only certain people to draw his blood or to do his procedures. I was one of the chosen few. Once when I was going to do a bone-marrow biopsy on him, his mother told me confidentially, "He trusts you. He knows you won't hurt him." That made me feel very nervous. I hoped he wasn't putting his trust in a person who might goof up. As I recall, that particular procedure went well. But it just as easily might not have gone so smoothly, and I wouldn't have forgiven myself easily.

Make-up, strong muscles, or a choice of doctors: anything that gave the children some sense of control over their frightening illnesses, which tossed them over precipices with no warning, helped them to cope.

Chapter 5

Carolina, Here I Come!

O for a beaker full of the warm South!

John Keats, "Ode to a Nightingale"

Phil and I had both paid for medical school through a state program that gave students money for promising to practice year for year in an underserved North Carolina community. So, after I had finished my residency in 1984, Phil and I wrote to the North Carolina rural board of health and asked them to send us names of all the rural areas in North Carolina that needed an internist and a pediatrician. At that point, Phil had a part-time job as an attending physician in the outpatient clinic at Hennepin County Medical Center, which allowed him to spend more time with our then almost two-year-old daughter, Ariel. I had been able to take six months out of my residency when she was born and then return.

We had a good response to our rural medicine search: fourteen communities were interested in talking to us. In a whirlwind two weeks, we visited all of them, my mother-in-law volunteering eagerly to keep Ariel during the day.

We ended up choosing Rutherford County, a community in the foothills of the Blue Ridge Mountains. My husband began with work at a multi-specialty clinic and I began part-time (though part-time for a doctor is still about 40 or more hours a week, if you include being on call) with a small pediatric group in town.

It was interesting, but it was very, very busy. There were nights when the phone would ring at 3 a.m. and one of us would answer it, sleepily asking, "Which doctor is it you want?"

Some of the late night/early morning phone calls would have been very funny if we hadn't been so tired. One mother called me to tell me, "I was biting off my baby's fingernails [a common custom in this area, though I didn't know that at the time] and I accidentally bit her finger. It looked okay when I put her to bed but now it's kind of red. Shall I bring her in to the Emergency Room?"

I assured her that it could wait until morning.

Another not uncommon call Phil and I would get went sort of like this:

"Hello. May I speak to the doctor? This is Harry Smith."

"I'm sorry. I don't remember the name. Can you tell me what the problem is?"

"I'm wheezing like crazy and I'm dizzy and my chest hurts. Dr. — told me to call whenever this happens."

"Oh so Dr. — is your doctor. Why didn't you call him?"

"Oh, I wouldn't want to wake him in the middle of the night!"

There were also the North Carolina mountain expressions and customs to learn. "High blood" means hypertension and "low blood" means anemia, so the doctor would be asked, "How can I have high blood and low blood at the same time?" "Infantigo" is an impetigo rash, which sort of made sense since it occurred mostly in babies. A "rising" or a "pone" is a boil and you "mash it" to remove it. You "mash" ganglion cysts with the largest book in the house, the family Bible. "Gouch" is gout, and "fireballs of the womb" are fibroid tumors. Elderly ladies used to go to the sheriff when they had a cough; he would mix them up some confiscated moonshine and some honey to control it. And many of them dipped snuff, which was considered more ladylike than smoking.

Our daughter Ariel was well behaved, and when we were both making rounds, she would sit and color happily at the nurses' station, enjoying candy and attention from the nurses. It wasn't easy, but it was manageable.

Then I took six months off with our second child, an exceptionally active boy, Alexander. He was another story altogether. I knew that I could not possibly handle what I was doing, and properly raise two children. As it was, at my partner's pleadings, I started back one afternoon a week when

Alex was two weeks old and had to interrupt my rushing from room to room to see patients in order to nurse him. A hungry baby does not take no for an answer.

Furthermore, there were some things about private practice that disappointed me. I never felt that I had enough time to spend with each patient. It was whip them in, and whip them out, so the doctor could see more of the long, forlorn line in the waiting room. I also found that, after working in my residency with children with very complex diseases, telling the twentieth mother of the day that, yes, her child did have the virus that was going around and that, no, there was very little to be done about it, I was looking for more variety.

I'm not putting down private pediatricians – not at all; it takes a skilled one to pick out the child with pneumonia or diabetes from the pack of mildly ill children and a very smart one to keep up with all the changes in treatment of so many different diseases. It was partly those types of decisions that kept me on edge and up in the night, hoping I had not made a mistake and going over and over what I had done. I suppose things would have improved over time. I hear my husband Phil giving instructions to the nurses over the phone while half asleep. He is so familiar with what to do in a certain situation that it is totally second nature, even if it is a crisis.

I got a call from a female pediatrician who had been in practice with her husband in various places in western North Carolina since the early 1950s.

"You may not be looking for another job," she said, "but I have six children and I remember what those days were like. There's a state-run developmental evaluation clinic in Morganton that needs a part-time doctor. Would you by any chance be interested?"

I could have kissed her feet.

I went to the interview with Alex in tow, since he was still nursing. I guess they figured I was knowledgeable about children.

I have been there ever since and, as my children have grown older, I have increased my time until I now work there four days a week, which gives me just enough time off still to keep the household running. In my opinion, I have one of the best doctor jobs available anywhere.

The State of North Carolina is unusual in that, since the 1970s, it has run 18 Developmental Evaluation Centers around the state. They are specifically intended for evaluating, diagnosing, and treating or finding treatment for children with a wide range of developmental and behavioral problems. The clinics are staffed by a doctor, a social worker, a psychologist, a speech and language pathologist, an educational diagnostician, a physical therapist, a nutritionist, and, more recently, an audiologist and an infant/toddler specialist. At our DEC we are fortunate to be friends as well as teammates.

Some or all of the specialists see each child who is referred, depending on what is needed, and then the group gets together to formulate a plan for the child and talk to the family. The benefits of this type of evaluation are that the team gets to spend a lot of time with the child and his or her family and that the child is viewed from many different perspectives.

If a child were brought in for a speech disorder, for example, our language therapists, Edie or Nadine, would be able to pinpoint the problems involved and how to treat him. She might wonder about a hearing disorder as well, and the audiologist would find a mild hearing loss. Our psychologist, Candace, would test the child's intelligence quotient (IQ) and figure out that the child was of normal intelligence, indicating that the language problem was a separate disability. The educational diagnostician, Wilson, would determine that the language problem was affecting the child's general knowledge and pre-academic skills and would decide what areas needed work.

I might discover that the child had a genetic syndrome causing that hearing loss. The physical therapist, Lela, would note that the child had balance difficulties. Lucy, our social worker, would pinpoint the stresses in the family that might interfere with their getting help for the child, and we would all brainstorm for solutions. Perhaps Lucy would discover that the family had no car to get the child to therapy appointments and would arrange for the family to get transportation.

That is just one example of how our team works. The people we serve come from all social classes, but the majority of them are poor.

Society is critical of the poor and the uneducated and so am I at times. I get awfully tired of the family that doesn't show for their appointment for the third time, or the father that smells so bad that we have to spray the office with air freshener after his visit, or the mother that doesn't follow through with the treatment that her child needs.

However, over time I've come to think of poor people as inexperienced jugglers trying to keep ten or twenty balls in the air. Perhaps the laundromat is closed, or the car breaks down, the sister who's helping out loses her job, the baby has a fever and no one can look after him, the father gets sent to jail for drug-dealing, the mother's jealous boyfriend calls Protective Services – and all the balls come falling down.

Being poor is no big deal when you know that you have a source of support standing guard in the background (like loving parents with deep pockets), such as I had during my medical school and residency. It is also no big deal if you know that you're working for something that will eventually lead you to financial comfort. It's the people who grew up in poverty, who are still living in poverty, and who never had the chance to escape poverty that have the most difficulty coping.

Money and education provide us with a backup that we can't begin to appreciate unless we know what it's like not to have them. That is why I feel angry when politicians insist that welfare mothers get jobs flipping burgers, forcing them to leave their children in substandard daycare.

I talked to a 20-year-old mother recently with two small children and a boyfriend, the father of both children, who is contributing no support to their care. She lives in a housing project. Her children get food stamps and Medicaid. However, their aid to federally dependent children has just been cut off. Why? The Work First program.

This is how it happened. She wants very much to get a job, but the community in which she lives is not hiring, they're laying off. She has no money to move. Furthermore, she was required to take part in Job Search, a requirement of Work First that involves spending several weeks job-hunting from 8 a.m. to 3 p.m. Because she had no one to keep her children, she could not attend. Because she did not attend, she was told that her children can no longer receive federal monies to help her care for them. Of course, the goal of Work First is admirable. If Work First provided quality daycare, this would not be a problem.

I should mention that the two girls were beautifully cared for, appropriately clothed, clean, and polite. Isn't that what we want mothers to be doing – raising happy and well-behaved children? Would we rather these two girls be in some home where they are plopped in front of a TV or not adequately supervised while their mother is still living in poverty despite her minimum-wage job?

Contrary to popular belief, parents on welfare have slightly fewer children (two) on average than the general population.[2] They are not baby factories. Furthermore, three-quarters of welfare recipients leave welfare within two years. Yes, this mother should not have gotten pregnant when she was 15. But she did. Are we going to punish her and her children for the rest of their lives? Unless we decide as a society to enforce contraception, force young girls to have abortions, or to give their babies up for adoption, the reality is that teenagers are going to have babies.

Once Candy, our nutritionist, and I were scheduled to make a home visit because the family had no transportation. They also had no phone. We called the number that had been given as a place to leave a message and there was no answer. We had sent them a letter telling them of the appointment, but there was no reply. We knew that the child badly needed to be seen: he had been scheduled before and had not shown up. Because of repeated requests from the Health Department and the child's primary doctor, we had rescheduled the child several times.

We decided to go and see if the family was home. We drove out to find a small trailer in the middle of nowhere. We knocked but there was no answer at all. When we drove off, we saw a light go on in the trailer. We felt frustrated and angry that someone had been there but had not bothered to let us in.

It turned out that the mother and child had fled an abusive father and were in hiding; a family friend was staying in their trailer. He had strict orders to let no one in and to call the police if the husband came, as a trespassing order had been taken out on him.

Eventually we did see the child. He had scars from where his father had beaten him with an electricity cord and his mother had two healing black eyes. I felt very bad for having been angry that they were "irresponsible" about keeping their appointment. What we see is only the tip of the iceberg for most of these families.

Chapter 6

Coping with a Disability

You grow up the day you have your first real laugh –
at yourself.

Ethel Barrymore

My first real experience with a child with multiple disabilities was when I was in seventh grade (aged 12). My friend Sandra had invited me to keep her company while she babysat for the day. She was watching a little girl, about five years old, who had multiple disabilities, including cerebral palsy, seizures, and profound mental retardation. I had never before been around a child with disabilities or heard much about them, and I was uncomfortable and frightened; terrified, actually. The child had a seizure while we were there, she spat and made funny noises, and when she was fed her baby food, she made a terrible mess. Sandra seemed to take it all in her stride. She had a cousin who had disabilities and babysat this child frequently. I marveled that she would be willing to watch the child and that she could stay so calm.

I laugh thinking about that day now because I clearly remember saying to myself when I went home, "I will never, never work with children like that when I grow up!" Life does throw some interesting curve balls.

Towards the end of my residency, I had a glimmer of what it was like to work with special children. I was doing a rotation in behavioral pediatrics and I arranged to attend testing once a week at Gillette Children's Hospital, for orthopedically handicapped children. The first child I saw tested was a little girl with Shirley Temple curls and beautiful blue eyes – and spastic quadriplegia, the type of cerebral palsy that causes stiffness and lack of coordination of the limbs as well as poor control of the neck, trunk, and mouth muscles. The child's family was from a very small town in South Dakota and they had done their best to take care of their daughter and include her in all the family activities, but had received no special therapies for her.

From looking at her, you would have thought she could do nothing. However, when the examiners took out the toys, you could see a gleam come into the little girl's eyes. With painstaking slowness, using her mouth and feet when they would help, she showed that she understood the tasks they were asking her to do. She found objects hidden under cups that had been shuffled around. She did puzzles. She matched common objects and pictures. She pointed to "the boy playing," "the girl having a drink."

Her parents had tears in their eyes when she was finished, and even the staff were moved. She herself seemed very triumphant. I realized that she wasn't unaware, just "locked in," kept from showing her active brain by her inability to move effectively. It was a real education for me. The parents were given information about how best to work with her and the names of agencies that could be helpful. They left the hospital feeling very proud of their daughter.

Children with disabilities are much more visible now than they were when I was growing up. Since their peers have been in preschool and school with them, see them on the bus, maybe help with Special Olympics, they grow up being more comfortable with differences in people in general. It is not in the least bit unusual to see an especially motherly kindergarten girl become the special friend of the child in the class with disabilities.

I see a little Mexican boy who has some learning problems, complicated by the fact that he still doesn't speak English well. Another Hispanic child in the class, Martina, who has lived in the United States longer and is very bright, has taken him under her wing. She sits beside him, helps him with his work, patiently translates what the teacher says, sits with him at lunch, and makes sure he is included in the games at recess. When I was asked what my recommendations were for the child, I replied, "Clone Martina!" I can think of a lot of other children who could use someone like her.

The attitude of more enlightened teachers has also made a big difference. What's more, with numerous kids going in and out of the main classroom for resource (remedial learning in a smaller setting), speech therapy, enrichment, occupational therapy, and social skills classes, another child with special needs coming and going becomes just another part of the day.

Sometimes, though, a child is not happy about being included in a regular curriculum. Danny was 15 when he decided to take charge of his life. He had leg deformities and was on crutches. He had extremely bad vision, even with thick glasses, and he was mildly hearing impaired. He had been diagnosed as educably mentally handicapped, which meant that his IQ was somewhere between 50 and 70.

I had seen Danny a number of times in the past and he struck me as a boy who never thought of himself as badly off. He had been in a foster-care home for many years, and his foster mother encouraged her foster children to be independent and adventuresome and to be their own advocates. She was certainly not the type to be at their beck and call. Nor did she show them pity and do things for them to compensate for their disabilities. She taught them to have backbone. I think some of the teachers cringed when they saw her coming, but she did get their respect.

Danny was in high school, in some special classes, but participating in physical education, lunch and some electives with the general program. He got very tired of being ridiculed and of having very few friends. He also wanted a girlfriend and saw no hope of that happening with the girls around him.

Danny had learned how to take the city bus by himself. One day, instead of going to high school, he got on the bus to a nearby town that had a special school for children with educational and other disabilities – though, in general, the children there had more learning problems than Danny. It is a wonderful school, colorful, with lots of specialized equipment, fun activities, and understanding teachers.

Danny went straight to the office.

"I'm here to go to this school," he announced. "I think I'll like it better here."

He had brought his school ID and he knew his address and telephone number. The secretary called his foster mother and she gave her permission for him to enroll. He had been talking to her about how he might want to go to this school.

Danny loved it there. As he was more intelligent than many of the children, he was a leader and sometimes a tutor. He was captain of the swimming team. He had loads of admiring friends. The teachers enjoyed his determination and his sense of humor. Because the kids got a lot of one-on-one attention, he also could learn at his level.

As he told everyone many times, to their surprised amusement at his sophistication, "That other school wasn't meeting my needs." I could tell that he was quoting his foster mother, but there was no doubt that he got the gist of what the phrase meant.

I still see Danny now and then. He is grown now and has a job he really enjoys, and he still shows the same grit and determination to work things out in his life and solve his problems on his own.

Chapter 7

Mental Retardation

People are like tea bags – you don't realize how strong they are until they get in hot water.

From a Salada tea bag

All right, none of us likes to be called dumb. No one wants to be called slow, learning impaired, dumb, educationally handicapped, but the really bad one is "mentally retarded." For many people, it brings forth images of drooling, screaming children in institutions. It is considered preferable in the UK to use the term "developmentally delayed" although the US still uses the term "mental retardation." Both are labels that, like so many other labels, cover a very wide range of different skill levels and characteristics.

The ICD-9, the diagnosis coding book (*International Classification of Diseases – Ninth Revision*), still includes words that used to be common for describing various levels of mental retardation such as idiot, imbecile, moron, and cretin. I only hope there are no doctors around who still use those words.

To be developmentally delayed does not mean a person can't learn. It doesn't mean a person will be in an institution. It doesn't even necessarily mean that the person is doomed always to live at home and never be able to hold a job. Not at all. In fact, we all probably have in our acquaintance several people who are technically mildly developmentally delayed. If we don't get into a conversation with them about anything more complicated than the weather or the local ball team, we won't know it. They function in society.

What developmentally delayed means is that, while a person with an average IQ (90–110) will make approximately one year's developmental and learning progress in one year's time during childhood, a person with developmental delay will make somewhere between one and seven months' progress in a year's time, depending on the severity of the mental retardation. In other words, if a child aged six is reasoning more like a child of four, and there are no external factors slowing his learning that can be corrected, then at age ten, he will probably be reasoning more like a child of six-and-a-half. He is making two-thirds of the progress that a child with an average IQ would make.

This does not mean that at age 40 the person will be functioning at a mental age of 26. He will not "catch up." But he will still be learning and acquiring new skills every day.

It is by no means easy to tell families bad news about their children, which is a large part of what we do at the DEC, but there is satisfaction in telling them in a sensitive and caring way. There is also a great deal of satisfaction in seeing that the children get the help they need and that the family gets the needed support. Most parents appreciate being told the truth, hard as it is to hear.

I have often heard a parent say about their four- or five-year-old child, "Why didn't someone tell us this before? We could have been doing something about it!" And they're right. Today it is being shown that early diagnosis and intervention prevent multiple problems later on – and saves society money, for that matter.

Mothers usually know there is something wrong. It is usually they who ask the doctor, "Shouldn't he be talking better by now?" They won't take a comforting pat on the shoulder for an answer. They want to know what is going on.

I know of one situation, in which the child not only turned out to be mentally retarded but also was found to have a dislocated hip, where the family physician answered the mother's concerned questions with, "Yes, he should be walking by now," and then walked out of the room without continuing the conversation. Obviously, that was not particularly helpful to her.

It seems to me that, although most fathers are very in touch with their children, if someone is going to be in denial, it is more commonly the father. Fathers are the ones who say, "There is nothing wrong with my child," much more often than mothers. Whether it is a macho thing or the fact that fathers are not usually the primary nurturers, I don't know. One father even threatened me by putting a fist in my face when I suggested his child had learning problems related to a disease called Albright syndrome, which, among other things, causes the fourth knuckle to dimple.

"Here," he said, thrusting his fist right up against my nose. "You just see if there's anything wrong with *my* knuckles!" I ducked out of the room, fast!

Some children with developmental delay never progress mentally beyond an infant stage, but this is the rarity. The main reason for having classifications of mild, moderate, severe, and profound developmental delay is so that children can get the services they need. In this world, a diagnosis is needed for insurance, for specialized services, for reimbursement programs, for school.

I don't like the phrase "mental retardation," but I have to use it. And it is important for parents to have a reasonable idea of what to expect for their child's future. It is usually one of the first questions they ask when they become aware that their child has a problem. The other two are, "Was this my fault?" and "What can we do now?"

Most professionals are also very careful to hold off giving a child the label of mental retardation until they are four or so and until they have been tested several times. Also, if anxiety, attention or behavior problems, language differences, or other physical disabilities such as visual impairment are affecting the testing, the scores should be interpreted with caution.

I have had personal experience of how stressful it is to have one's child tested and also how behavior can affect a test score. I remember when Ariel was tested to see if she was ready for kindergarten. She did "pass," but in the car on the way back home, she told me, "They asked me where my nose was, and I did this!" (pointing to her eye). "Wasn't that a funny joke, Mama?"

Yes, Ariel, very funny. I'm laughing hysterically.

There are times when a child can seem to be developmentally delayed, but there is a medical cause behind it. Melissa was 12 when she was brought in by her school guidance counselor to be tested. She was there because she had been doing terribly in school for two years. Prior to that she had been a poor student but nowhere near as confused and slow as she was by the time I saw her.

Her guidance counselor was not the most sensitive of people.

"Now Melissa, you sit right here and wait for me to talk to the doctor," she said loudly and slowly. Then she walked about three feet away to talk to me.

"I want you to see if she's anemic. She never has any energy and she's always complaining about feeling bad. Of course, I don't know what else you could expect. Her mother doesn't ever communicate with the school even though we send her notes all the time. Melissa is always sleeping in class. I don't how late she's allowed to stay up. I think Melissa is…" She looked back at Melissa and then turned to me and stage-whispered, "mentally retarded."

I tried to stop the flow of words and smiled at Melissa encouragingly. After introducing myself, I took her back to my office.

Melissa was a short and plump child who had not yet started puberty. Her face was puffy and she did have something of a dull look in her eyes. She was wearing a fuzzy sweater even though it was summer. She tended to look down at the floor. When I closed the door to my office, she looked at me seriously and said in a surprisingly husky voice,

"I don't know what's wrong with me. I can't do well at school anymore. If I am mentally retarded, please let me know because I need to learn how to cope with it."

Well, that speech gave me a clue right away that there was more to Melissa than met the eye. Most 12-year-old children with developmental delay – or for that matter, without it! – would not have such a clear under-standing of their plight or the maturity to discuss their problems so candidly.

I examined Melissa. Her skin was dry with scaly patches and a sallow color. Her hair was thin and brittle. Her deep tendon reflexes were slow. She seemed to have difficulty with her balance and coordination. I asked her if she had trouble with constipation and she told me that she did. Most impor-tantly, she had a goiter – an enlarged thyroid.

"Am I retarded?" she asked me, again.

"We haven't tested you, but I really don't think so," I told her. "I think you have something wrong with your thyroid that is making you very tired. We're going to need to do some blood tests on you."

As I had expected, Melissa's testing showed that she was hypothyroid. She saw an endocrinologist, began to take an artificial thyroid hormone,

Synthroid, and became a changed child. She grew several inches and began to develop breasts and hips. Her face lost its dull look. She joined the basketball team. Though she was never a top student, her schoolwork improved markedly. No one ever again wondered whether she was mentally retarded.

There is another situation in which children can appear mentally retarded when their potential is far beyond that. A delayed child just removed from a neglectful situation may improve by leaps and almost miraculously in a new environment.

We saw a three-year-old boy, Jamal, who went to live with loving foster parents after having been abused and neglected by his cocaine-addicted mother and her various boyfriends. He had been left in a playpen most of the time as a baby and as he grew older had been cared for by one stranger after another – whoever his mother could get to keep him for a few days. He hadn't had enough food and was still on the bottle at three. He had terrible "bottle rot" teeth. There were cigarette burns on his arms and several unexplained scars. He was still in diapers and had a bad rash from being very infrequently changed. He was terribly thin and his dark skin had an ashy gray tint.

Jamal could hardly talk when we saw him, a month after his having been put in foster care. He was withdrawn and seemed almost autistic-like in his avoidance of interaction. He screamed when he was upset, he bit his hands, and banged his head. He was very underweight and when he was given food, he often hid it under his bed, acting as if he did not know when he would get to eat next (not surprising, under the circumstances). He came across as quite developmentally delayed and, sure enough, he tested more like a 15-month-old.

His foster parents were patient and gave him love, gentle discipline, and plenty of learning opportunities. He received speech therapy. His foster brothers and sisters, who were older, all fussed over him, giving him piggyback rides and having wrestling matches with him (which Jamal usually "won").

When we saw Jamal a year later, he was a stocky and handsome little guy who was hardly recognizable as the waif we had seen the year before. He talked in full sentences and initiated a game with the other child in the waiting room. He loved to look at books and be read to. He ran down the hall holding hands with the educational diagnostician and gladly accepted stickers for good work. He sang us his favorite TV commercials. His repeat testing by our psychologist, Candace, came out in the low average range, more like a three-and-a-half year old. He had made 27 months' progress in a year's time! His foster parents were in the process of adopting him.

"If you change your minds, we'll take him," we told them.

The mother shook her head, laughing. "Not in a million years," she said.

Jamal was one of the lucky ones. In fact, many children who have been neglected in their first few years never fully recover. Inadequate nutrition and poor parenting can cause the brain to be 20 to 30 percent smaller than average. An adult's final vocabulary can be predicted by verbal abilities at age three and their math and logic abilities can be predicted by age four. Babies are born with about one billion brain cells and as young children learn from their environment, the brain cells begin to form connections and new cells are made. Eventually in adulthood, there can be as many as one thousand trillion cells. However, the growth of the brain is directly related to learning experiences, and most of them make connections and grow in the first few years of life.[3, 4]

Children who have not formed a bond with a nurturing adult by age three can fail ever to exhibit the normal development of empathy. They have trouble forming meaningful relationships. We sometimes see this show up in the opposite way than you might expect. Sometimes a child who has just been removed from a situation of abuse or neglect will come running up to you, crawl all over you, hug and kiss you, not want to leave. Starved for attention? Yes, such children are also unable to distinguish between the love of an adult who knows them well and cares for them and the less personal kindness of a stranger. These children are at risk of being sexually abused. They are also very easily influenced by peer pressure. They often have nightmares and other signs of deep anxiety. This is called an "attachment disorder."

There are worse things than being developmentally delayed. Being unable to trust and to love in an appropriate way is a far more serious handicap for a happy and successful life. Nevertheless, I understand why most parents are stricken when we have to tell them that their child is retarded.

We currently care for a child with a chromosomal disorder that is known to cause developmental delay, and the parents refuse to acknowledge that there is anything wrong with their six-year-old who talks in single words and is not yet toilet trained. They insist that he will be going to college. I feel great sympathy for them, but their unwillingness to accept their child's disability is clearly not in the child's best interest. As we say at the DEC, "Denial is not just a river in Egypt."

On the other hand, we once told a mother, who had been obliging and friendly but had had trouble answering our questions, the news that her child was developmentally delayed. A light came into her eyes.

"Oh, okay," she said. "I'm mentally retarded. I know what that is."

She realized that this was something she could deal with.

I enjoy going to the Down Syndrome Association's yearly conferences in Charlotte because it is a wonderful opportunity to see how families and children have coped with their special situations. One family told the audience about their 15-year-old son, David, who had fallen in love with a girl, Jennifer, in his special education class, and she with him. They held each other's hands and spent every moment at school together. When at home, they talked to each other on the phone for hours.

"I'm going to marry Jennifer," David said frequently. His parents smiled indulgently. When he was younger, he had told them that he was going to be a pro football player, too.

Both sets of parents assumed that it was puppy love and several years later, when the girl's father was transferred to another town, they said, "Well, that's the end of that."

But it wasn't. The young adults continued to stay in contact and David continued to insist that he loved Jennifer. When Jennifer came with her family for a visit, she and David ran to each other and held each other in a long, ecstatic embrace.

"When I saw their faces, I knew that I couldn't keep fighting the inevitable," said David's mother. Jennifer's parents were concerned, but the families got together and discussed all the potential solutions and their ramifications.

David and Jennifer were married in a happy ceremony attended by many friends and two big families. They made up their own vows. They spent their honeymoon in a suite in the Blue Ridge Mountains with Jennifer's parents staying next door. Now the newlywed couple lives with David's family. They have their own separate quarters in the basement. Both of them work at jobs in the community, David with a lawn service and Jennifer at a grocery store. They are as happy as any young married couple can be. Their parents know they made the right decision.

Another young woman in her thirties with Down syndrome told about her decision to live on her own. After much argument and discussion, she convinced her family that this was the right thing for her. She knows how to take the bus to her job and she can cook for herself. Relatives check on her regularly and she also has a social worker who makes sure she is doing fine.

Someone asked her how her mother felt about her living alone.

"She was pretty worried at first," said the young woman, smiling indulgently. "But, you know, that's how mothers are."

Chapter 8

Genetics and Syndromes

There never were in the world two opinions
alike, no more then two hairs or two grains;
the most universal quality is diversity.

Michel de Montaigne

I spent my preschool and elementary school years in Puerto Rico because of
my father's job in industrial relations that sent him all over the world. It was
a wonderful place to grow up. Our neighborhood in Old San Juan was a
mixture of houses restored by the wealthy and middle class and old build-
ings with peeling paint and plaster. Some of my friends were picked up from
school in limousines and others walked home in cheap *choncletas*, rubber
sandals that could be purchased at the five-and-dime store.

I knew very little about racial prejudice. There were Puerto Ricans with
skin that ranged from the palest ivory to the darkest black, and everything in
between: too many shades of brown to distinguish between. The people
who looked really strange to me were the US tourists who came every
winter to enjoy the sun. I remember thinking to myself, "Why are their
bodies so pasty white all over?" and "Why do they want to lie in the sun until
they turn red?" By the time I had lived in Canada a few years, when we
followed my father's job to British Columbia (where I spent my high school
years), I had more sympathy for pasty white people. In fact, I had a sneaking
suspicion that I was one myself.

Thanks to the diversity of Puerto Rico, I was used to differences in body type and skin color. However, all children are curious about what they have never seen before. As a little girl, I remember the first time I saw a child with Down syndrome. I was playing in the park. There were several mango trees in the playground, and we boys and girls used to throw rocks at the mangos, hoping that they would fall to the ground so we could share the sweet, sticky fruit with our best friends. We ran, jumped rope, and played four-square, basketball, and hopscotch.

One morning there was a little boy there, holding hands with his mother and watching us from the side. I knew there was something different about him by his unusual appearance and even by the loose-jointed way that he walked. I went over to the bench where my parents were sitting and tugged on my father's arm until he bent over.

"What's wrong with that boy?" I whispered.

"He's a Mongoloid," my father told me. That was what everyone called children with Down syndrome then because of their slanted eyes. It's a major misnomer, since children who really are Mongolian and have Down syndrome are very readily identifiable as different from others of their ethnic origin. Actually, I myself have slightly slanted eyes because of my Russian ancestry, and I sure don't think I look like I have Down syndrome!

What are you doing when you look at a person and know automatically that he or she has Down syndrome? Though you may not realize it, your mind is going through the following analytic process: small person, boxy head and stocky body, upslanting eyes, tongue looks large, short hands and fingers – must be someone with Down syndrome.

That is exactly what doctors do when they are trying to make a diagnosis. It's like putting a puzzle together. First you analyze the individual pieces, then you see how they fit together, then you see the whole. I always have a feeling of excitement and challenge when I get a new jigsaw puzzle and lay out all the pieces on the table. I enjoy diagnosing genetic syndromes for the same reason.

The word "syndrome" means a group of symptoms that are found together frequently enough that they can be grouped under one name. The physical and clinical features of syndromes often come from the same genetic or environmental causes, but not always.

The reason it is important to determine whether a child has a syndrome is to make sure that he or she does not have other hidden problems that often go with the same diagnosis. Also, some syndromes are treatable, and some can be inherited by future generations.

If a doctor becomes familiar with the symptoms of a particular syndrome, especially if it's relatively unusual, then he or she can look like a wizard to a patient's parents.

I once had a mother bring in her 12-month-old who was severely hearing impaired. They could not find a cause for the hearing impairment and wondered whether it might be related to a fever of 104°F he had at six months of age. Contrary to popular belief, a fever must be very, very high – 107°, 108°F or more – and prolonged if it is going to cause brain damage. I knew his fever was unlikely to be the cause of the child's deafness.

I watched the child as he played with the psychologist. He was somehow familiar looking. He resembled his mother but it was more than that. He had a very wide jaw and really strikingly blue eyes. His eyes were very wide-spaced and his eyebrows flared in the middle. His nose dipped a little lower in the center than on the sides.

"You might think I'm crazy, but does anyone in your family have a white patch of hair right above the middle of his forehead?" I asked, suddenly.

She stared at me, her mouth open in shock.

"How in the world did you know that?" she asked, wonderingly. "My dad does. He's had it since he was a little boy."

"I know what is causing your son's deafness. He has Waardenburg syndrome," I told her. "It wasn't the high fever."

That may sound impressive. But to people that frequently work with children with profound deafness, it's pretty much like a mechanic being able to tell you why your car isn't running. It's not common, but common enough that most teachers of the deaf see several children with Waardenburg syndrome in their career.

Waardenburg syndrome is one of those genetic groupings of symptoms that includes nerve deafness, wide jaws and wide-spaced eyes, and pigment changes that can cause very blue eyes, white forelocks and white patches on the skin.[5] Like many other syndromes, it has "variable penetrance," meaning that even within the same family, some people can have only a very few of the symptoms and some can have all of them. In this case, the grandfather had the partial pigment loss, the mother had some of the typical facial features and the child had the whole syndrome.

I saw another child with the same syndrome, Waardenburg's, whose parents were claiming that he had been made deaf by an immunization during infancy. North Carolina offers compensation for children damaged by state-required vaccines, so there was money in the diagnosis.

This child did not have all the symptoms, but, again, she gave me that "I know what this is; it's on the tip of my tongue" feeling. She did have the deafness. She had the wide-spaced eyes and the wide jaw. She did not have pigmentary changes such as the white forelock, and her eyes were hazel, though slightly different from each other in color.

After a lot of deliberation, I told them I thought that the reason for her deafness was that she had Waardenburg syndrome. They denied that this was the case; they were sure that she had been able to hear when she was born, which would be impossible with this syndrome. They insisted that she was deaf because of the vaccine.

I happened to be talking about this child to a psychologist colleague who had tested her a month before. He readily agreed that the child had Waardenburg's.

"Sure, that's what I thought she had, too," he said. "Didn't you see her white forelock?"

I later found out that the parents had already been to a geneticist who told them that their daughter had Waardenburg syndrome, but they didn't like what they heard, since the vaccine-injuries program wouldn't pay for that. So apparently they decided to either dye or cut out the white patch of hair, comb over the spot, and take her to another doctor. I don't know this for a fact, but the white forelock was certainly not there when I saw the child. They may still have been convinced that the vaccine had caused the problem, for all I know. People can be very good at believing what they want to believe.

When I told the state's lawyer about all of this, the case was quickly settled out of court.

The most common syndrome and the most common cause of mental retardation is not Down syndrome. It's not even genetic. It's something that could be prevented in every case. It is fetal alcohol syndrome.

Of every thousand children born in the United States, between one and three has fetal alcohol syndrome, and at least twice that many children have some of the symptoms and effects of alcohol exposure while in the womb. Children with fetal alcohol syndrome have many problems beyond learning difficulties. They often have hyperactivity, behavior problems and hearing deficits. They have particular trouble with math and nonverbal tasks. They may also have difficulty in recording, processing, interpreting and using information.[6]

This is a subtle syndrome, with a higher index of suspicion if it is known that the mother used alcohol to excess. The children are small and have small heads. Their eyes are small, with a fold at the inner corner, and the eyelids may droop. The distance between the nose and mouth is increased and the little scoop between them, called the philtrum, is absent. The top of the lip often does not have the little cupid's bow and the red part is thin. They can have heart disease, cleft lip and palate, and many other problems.

We think of cocaine as being a very dangerous drug and, of course, it is. But short of the severe damage cocaine can do to a developing fetus, such as strokes and missing limbs, alcohol is much more poisonous. Children who have been exposed to cocaine in the womb usually have minimal problems if they are removed from the home of cocaine-addicted parents who have nothing else on their minds but getting their next high. In fact a study done by Dr. Deborah Frank and her colleagues suggests that many of the problems children have that were attributed to cocaine use actually have more to do with concurrent use of tobacco, marijuana and alcohol.[7]

Children of alcoholic mothers are not so lucky – the damage is already done. We have seen several children who were adopted who were later discovered to have fetal alcohol syndrome. Even more tragic is when the mother has recovered from alcoholism, is sober, and knows what she did to her child.

I know one mother, a former drinker, who has a child with fetal alcohol syndrome. When we saw her child, he was seven and in his second year of kindergarten. Although friendly and likeable, he was extremely active, climbing under tables, turning flips down the hall and ripping the pillows off the rocking chair. We certainly had no worries about his large muscle skills!

Finally, Lucy, our social worker, stopped him and held him in her lap. Nicky wriggled and squirmed for a while, but then settled in to cuddle. "I think he's going to give me a heart attack," she told the mother. "Tell me about it," said his mother wearily. "That's what my life is like."

The boy, Nicky, had been born weighing three pounds, even though he was full term. He had always been tiny and had been a very fussy and difficult feeder through the first year of life. His mother spent a lot of nights walking the floor with him.

His physical exam showed that he had some of the features I previously described, including the thin upper lip, a small head, eye folds, curved fifth fingers and difficulty fully turning his forearms back and forth or hands up and hands down. He was of borderline to low average intelligence, but with a marked weakness in his abilities to do mazes, puzzles, block design and other performance items. And as we determined from observation, questionnaires, and the mother's and teacher's reports, he did have attention deficit hyperactivity disorder.

I asked, as I always do, about alcohol consumption during pregnancy. She told me that she had drunk about two beers a day. I asked her about any binge drinking and she denied this. She did admit to smoking two packs of cigarettes, as well. Actually, cigarette smoking is the most common reason for a low birthweight baby, so the combination of smoking and drinking is especially bad.

I do not know if she was markedly underestimating her drinking during pregnancy (which is likely) or if she was just very unlucky. We do not really know how much alcohol is safe during pregnancy and at what specific point during the pregnancy it is the most dangerous, though some studies would indicate that it takes about three drinks a day to cause significant harm.

The other reason I suspected that she was not telling the truth about how much she drank is that the school reported that she had been seen intoxicated at school when picking up Nicky.

When we told her that her child probably had fetal alcohol syndrome, she cried and cried.

"This is my fault, then?" She put her head down on the table. I sat beside her, helpless, one hand on her shoulder.

"Do you want me to leave you alone for a few minutes and then come back?"

She nodded. I left, closing the door behind me and taking some deep breaths to compose myself, too.

It is very hard being the bearer of bad news but especially hard when the person you are telling is responsible for the tragedy. Parents always worry that their children's problems relate to something they did wrong, and in this case, it was true. I did tell her not to blame herself too much, because addiction is a very difficult problem to overcome, and I knew she would not deliberately have hurt her baby. We encouraged her to go to Alcoholics Anonymous or to see a counselor. She found the strength to do this, though she worried to us that she would get in trouble with the law for having damaged her child.

She has been sober for four years now and devotes a good bit of time to teaching others about the problem and counseling pregnant women who are drinking. She still carries around an enormous burden of guilt, though she realizes that alcoholism is a disease and that she had little control over her behavior at the time. She hopes that the lesson she learned the hard way can be used to help others. I feel that what she does takes great courage, not just to stay sober but to use her misfortune in a positive way.

A syndrome that I find particularly interesting is Williams syndrome. The children who have this are adorable; in fact, many syndromes do not make the afflicted child unattractive. These children look like little elves. They have heart-shaped faces, a starlike pattern in their irises, upturned little noses, and wide mouths. They are generally very small. They also frequently have heart disease, particularly a type where the aorta is narrowed and the blood pressure is very high, which is the most life-threatening part of the syndrome.

What is interesting about children with Williams syndrome is that their personalities are very similar.[8] They are almost all quite friendly and verbal, chattery, in fact, and excel at reading as compared to other children at their intellectual level (the syndrome does cause developmental delay, with an average IQ of 50–70). They often love music and literature. However, their ability to organize material and listen to language, their visual-spatial skills, and their drawing abilities are disastrous. Their drawings may have a lot of detail, but are completely disorganized, with pieces of the drawing all over the page and no coherent whole.

The main chemical abnormality that is found in these children is an elevated calcium level at birth, and it may be that there is an underlying defect in the way the body handles calcium. This could definitely affect the development of the brain, since it regulates the release of calcium from the cells.

In *Discovery* magazine, the writer, Eleanor Semel, describes these children. "Educators are confused because the Williams syndrome child tests like a retarded child, talks like a gifted child, behaves like a disturbed child, and functions like a learning-disabled child."[9] Clearly, such children are hard to educate.

I find these peaks and valleys in ability interesting because this small chromosomal change that we can now test for in these children is not only producing physical symptoms but also affecting specific areas of their brains. This brings up all sorts of questions about genetic differences and various specific learning disabilities in children who are otherwise quite capable.

Children with Williams syndrome almost all tend to be hypersensitive to noise. I knew one patient, Chip, who kept crying one summer every time he went outside. His family knew that he disliked things like vacuum cleaners and lawn mowers, but they didn't know what was bothering him this time. Then they realized that it was one of the 17-year locust birth cycles and that the high-pitched, throbbing chirps of the insects that they just filtered out were driving the poor child crazy.

On the other hand, his favorite thing to do was to sit quietly by the stereo and listen to Bach. When his preschool teacher asked each child to bring a recording of his favorite song, Chip brought Pachelbel's *Canon in D*. Chip is a teenager by now and I doubt very much that he is spending his allowance on rap CDs! He has probably widened his horizons to Debussy or Gregorian Chants.

Now for a *Jeopardy* question: what is the commonest inherited type of mental retardation? (By inherited, I mean that it is not just a gene abnormality that occurs randomly, but one that is passed on in families.)

To answer in proper Alex Trebek style: "What: is Fragile X syndrome?"

Many people haven't heard of it, and it creates only very subtle physical differences in a child. These can include long faces, large ears that often stick out, prominent foreheads and jaws, hyperflexible joints, chests that cave in, and – as generally only boys with this syndrome reach puberty – testicles that are much larger than normal. To complicate matters further, some children who have it (and have the associated learning or behavior problems) look completely normal.[10]

The rule of thumb given to doctors is that if there is unexplained mental retardation in a child who has a family with a history of developmental delay, do the blood test for Fragile X. Some doctors even test anyone with an unexplained developmental delay.

I used to see a delightful family with a child, Damone, who was severely retarded because his mother had been exposed to toxoplasmosis, a virus sometimes found in cat feces, while she was pregnant. (This is an excellent reason to get one's husband to change the litter box if one is pregnant!) Damone was an exceptionally sweet child with a smile and a laugh for everyone, and I always enjoyed his visits. He was somewhat different-looking; as well as a small head, he had huge sticking-out ears and a large jaw. Of course, we had the reason for his mental retardation already determined, so we looked no further. Doctors, including myself, told his mother that she would have no risk of having another baby affected by toxoplasmosis.

So they had Tyrique. Tyrique, though far more capable than Damone, also had learning problems, and he was hyperactive and very shy, giving very poor eye contact. He frequently bit his hands and had calluses on them. He had protruding ears, a prominent forehead and jaw, hyperflexible joints – and when we tested him, we discovered that he had Fragile X syndrome. So we tested Damone and discovered that he had it, too – but I had never suspected it.

From a genetic viewpoint, Fragile X is one of the most interesting of chromosomal abnormalities. It is X-linked, meaning that it is passed on through the mother's X chromosome. Diseases that are X-linked either affect girls less severely, or not at all (though they are carriers), because they have one normal X to protect and mask the abnormal X. Boys, who are XY and only have one X, are far more affected if the X is an abnormal one. Other examples of X-linked diseases are most forms of color blindness and Duchenne's muscular dystrophy.

Fragile X syndrome is also fascinating because it worsens with each generation. It is caused by a piece of the X chromosome that repeats and repeats its DNA message. Interestingly enough, we have discovered that a lot of our chromosomal material is "filler" or "nonsense" material, and all of us have repeating patterns in all our chromosomes. However, if a person has too many repeats in this particular area on the X chromosome, he has Fragile X. In each successive generation, the number of repeats gets worse, and the larger the number of repeats, the worse the symptoms are.

Sometimes when we delve into a family tree we discover that there is a generation with no learning problems, then a generation where several of the children had some minor learning problems, such as difficulties with math computation and comprehension. Finally there comes the child in the third generation with the full-blown Fragile X syndrome.

I see another family with two Fragile X children. The parents have no learning problems at all and even have one daughter who excels at schoolwork and art. The Fragile X boy, however, has mild mental retardation, a diagnosis of mild autism, and some behavior problems which are managed well with Adderal (a stimulant) and Paxil (an antidepressant and antianxiety medication). The Fragile X daughter has some learning problems in math and written language and poor social skills. When I first met her, she would respond to everything I said with, "That's utterly ridiculous!" She was also very shy, though she has gradually outgrown this. Both children have a secondary diagnosis of attention deficit hyperactivity disorder, which is another symptom of Fragile X.

They are now teenagers and doing well. Nathan is reading well and has discovered soccer. Amanda is making lots of friends and has a part-time job. At some point Amanda needs to be told that she has a 50 percent chance of having a daughter who has Fragile X or who is a carrier and a 50 percent chance of having a son with Fragile X. Nathan, on the other hand, would have all normal boys, since the father provides the Y and not the X to his sons, and all his girls would have Fragile X or be carriers. It's surprisingly complicated.

The two most extraordinary syndromes from a standpoint of new information about genetics are Prader-Willi and Angelman: syndromes with totally different symptoms that are both caused by the same chromosomal defect.[11] Prader-Willi is associated with very low muscle tone in infancy, small size, small feet, small head, developmental delay, and later obesity with an uncontrolled appetite – quite often even for non-foods. Once I was drawing blood from a child with Prader-Willi, and while I turned my head momentarily to grab a Bandaid, she put the test tube in her mouth.

Angelman syndrome is associated with a big lower jaw and a small upper jaw, light-colored eyes and hair, a large mouth, wide-spaced teeth, jerky movements, and developmental delay. What is so bizarre is that if the defective chromosome comes from the mother, the child has Angelman syndrome. If it comes from the father, the child has Prader-Willi syndrome.

And yet we have no idea why this makes a difference, since all our chromosomal material is randomly selected from either our father or our mother! Do the same "Mama" and "Daddy" chromosomes actually have different functions within the cell? And if so, what does this mean in terms of the effects of those random "Mama" and "Daddy" combinations on all of us?

How do you tell a boy chromosome from a girl chromosome? You pull down its "genes." That joke's been around for a long time but the question may actually make some scientific sense.

As the human genome project and the continuing analysis of our chromosomal material continues, we will have more and more of the answers to these questions. I find it very exciting.

Chapter 9

Sandra's Story

"But see here!" said Jack Pumpkinhead, with a gasp: "if you become a girl, you can't be my dear father anymore!"
"No," answered Tip, laughing in spite of his anxiety; "and I will not be sorry to escape the relationship." Then he added, hesitatingly, as he turned to Glinda: "I might try it for awhile, just to see how it seems, you know. But if I don't like being a girl you must promise me to change me into a boy again."

L. Frank Baum, The Land of Oz

For anyone who questions whether the world has become a better place for people who are different, I will tell Sandra's story.

When Sandra's mother gave birth to her, no one cried out joyfully, "It's a boy!" or "It's a girl!" There was silence in the delivery room. Sandra had what is called, in medical terminology, "ambiguous genitalia." She also had some other minor malformations such as an extra toe on each foot, a curved leg, and a malformed kidney that later needed to be removed.

Ambiguous genitalia – in other words, genitals that are somewhere between those of a male and a female – can occur for various reasons. Frequently, there has been a hormonal abnormality in the womb. For example, when a baby girl's adrenal hormones are not properly balanced, the hormones can act like testosterone and cause the clitoris to grow more like a small penis. The labia may fuse shut, resembling empty scrotal sacs. The child also has trouble retaining salt and may have some increased pigmentation. All of this is due to hormonal imbalance and it can be corrected for the child's health. The decision that needs to be made with all children with ambiguous genitalia is whether it is wiser to raise them as a boy or a girl. This is not always determined by what their chromosomes indicate they are. Sometimes it depends on how much surgery must be done to make them look more like one or the other.

As if that weren't a difficult enough decision for the parents to make, at the same time, they are facing what to tell the outside world. What have they named the baby? Is it a boy or a girl? Why is it still in the hospital? Parents are frequently advised to tell everyone except close family members that the baby is sick and must remain in the hospital for a while and that they don't feel they can discuss it further at that time.

This baby's chromosomes and hormones were checked, and it was determined that "it" was chromosomally a male. However, its genitalia appeared much more female and after a good bit of discussion among doctors and the family, it was decided to raise the baby as a girl. Some minor corrective surgery would be done and eventually, when she was older, the testicles that were still high up in her body like ovaries would be removed. Naturally, she could never have children.

So the baby had the extra toes removed, a cast placed on the curved leg, and left the hospital in a beautiful pink sleeper, bundled into a car seat for her ride home. She was christened Sandra. Her whole family loved her without reservation and she became a sturdy baby and then an active toddler. Sandra's family was smart, though. As soon as she was old enough to understand some of what they were telling her, they told her a little bit about her birth. The little girl with the curly golden hair past her waist knew from an early age that the reason she had to have some surgeries along the way and frequently had to be checked for other problems was because she had some big differences about her body.

As we continued to follow Sandra, her mother expressed some minor concerns. Sandra was something of a tomboy. She loved to play with cars and trucks, enjoyed rough and tumble play in the backyard with her father and brothers, and was highly active. I was not worried.

"Lots of little girls are tomboys," I said. "It often means that they will be capable, independent women."

Kindergarten came. Sandra continued to be the energetic and curious child she had always been. She loved the water table and the housekeeping center and, most of all, the sports the children played outside at lunch and recess. She could throw a ball more accurately than anyone else in the class. She won a number of ribbons on Field Day for running the fastest. Her father was called to school one day to pick her up when she and a boy in her class had gotten into a brief tussle. Sandra seemed proud of her black eye.

First grade came and went. Then, in second grade, Sandra dropped her bombshell.

"Mama, Daddy, I have something to tell you," she said one day at the dinner table. "I am a boy. I have always felt like a boy. I want to be a boy."

Her parents were stunned. They didn't know what to do. Sandra was the only granddaughter. They dressed her in smocked and frilly dresses on Sundays. She and her mother had their special Saturdays together when they went and had their nails manicured. And now she was telling them that she wasn't a girl; she was a boy. And, of course, they knew that, technically, she was right. This was despite the fact that they had never actually told her that she was chromosomally XY.

So they made some phone calls and drove to a large city in a neighboring state where they had heard there was an excellent psychiatrist who specialized in gender identity.

Sandra and the psychiatrist met together for two or three hours. Sandra was her usual friendly, emphatic self and she told the psychiatrist all about her life. At the end of the time, they came out to talk to her parents.

"There's no doubt about it," the psychiatrist said. "Sandra is a boy."

So how did Sandra's parents handle this revelation? They sensibly decided that she was, in fact, a boy. They cut her hair in a short boyish cut, they started dressing her in her favorite T-shirts and jeans, and they talked to the doctors about changing the surgery planned for the future. They knew it meant more hospitalizations, but they also realized it was the only way for Sandra to live a full and successful life.

Sandra and her mother went to school to talk to her teacher and principal at length. The next morning, Sandra's mother stayed at the beginning of class.

"Boys and girls," said the teacher, "Sandra has something to tell us."

A child, looking very much like Sandra's older brother, came up. It was Sandra! The child smiled at the class and began talking.

"I used to dress like a girl," she told them. "But I'm not. I'm a boy and my name is Sandy. My dad's name is Alexander and now I'm named after him." Sandy's mother stood beside him.

"Does anyone have any questions?" she asked.

Hands shot up all over the place. The children were fascinated, and there was a good bit of giggling, but they were not disgusted or horrified.

"Are you going to change your last name, too?"

"What does Max think? Does he like having another brother?"

"Who cut your hair?"

"Are you going to have a wee-wee?"

"Will you pee sitting down or standing up?"

Sandy and her mother and teacher answered the questions as best they could. The class talked for a long time. Finally the questions died down. Sandy went and sat down in his usual seat. His best friend, Jonathan, punched his arm playfully.

It is now a year later. Sandy has lots of friends at school and is in the Cub Scouts. Grown-ups do often whisper behind his back, but most of the children don't. They know Sandy is the same person they've known since kindergarten.

The most amazing thing about the whole story is that Sandy is a happy and confident child. Wilson, the educational diagnostician at the DEC, who has spent a lot of time with Sandy, remarked that he thought that Sandy was one of the most well-adjusted children he knew.

He still has some major surgery in store and a penis to be constructed. However, everyone knows that Sandy is on his way. And he is still the best four-square player in his class.

Chapter 10

Learning Disabilities

I never let my schooling interfere with my education.

Mark Twain

My mother was a school librarian. The most exciting part of the summer was when the new books that she had ordered for her library arrived. My sister Kim and I had the honor of opening the boxes, smelling that wonderful new-book smell, and choosing the ones we wanted to read before school started. I can remember spending hours lying on the cold marble floor, with the ceiling fan blowing full blast, reading book after book in the heat of a Puerto Rican summer day.

I can't imagine what it would be like not to be able to read. Reading has always been an integral part of my life, first being read to and then reading to myself. I can't get through a day without a little time to read. It's sort of like breathing to me. I carry a book everywhere I go, even to the checkout counter at the grocery store.

And yet I see children all the time who struggle with reading no matter how hard they work at it. They would rather dig ditches than fight their way through a book, especially if they have to read aloud in front of their class.

There was a boy in my elementary-school classes who loved to draw. He wasn't very interested in school or very good at it, and most of the day, while the teacher talked, he drew in his notebook. But what drawings! They were amazingly well done for a child of his age. Scuba divers, surfers, soldiers, horses – he could really make things come alive with just a pencil and an 11

61

x 14 standard piece of ruled paper. We would stand around and tell him what we wanted him to draw.

"Make a tiger." And a tiger would seem magically to appear out of his pencil.

"Draw Mrs. Diaz." And there was a wickedly accurate caricature of our teacher.

I was always fascinated by what he could do. The art teacher loved him, but the rest of the teachers got very irritated with his poor grades and inattention. He was sent out to the hall a lot – standard punishment in those days, but pretty dumb, really, for a child who already isn't paying attention to schoolwork. It's like making an overly fidgety child miss recess.

Today, I understand, he is a very successful graphic artist. I'm not surprised.

The true definition of a learning disabled individual is a person with normal intelligence, who may, in fact, excel in some areas but who has one or more areas of learning which do not come at all naturally to him or her.

Most of us have an area for which this is true. I, for example, have no sense of direction and have to rely on maps and written instructions to get anywhere, often even if I'm headed there for the second or third time. However, since I'm not part of a nomadic culture where finding my way is the most essential skill needed in life, I am not considered stupid. It is when the child's disability is in a field taught at school that the trouble begins.

The public school's definition of a learning disability is when a child scores 15 or more points lower than their measured IQ in an area like reading, math, or written expression. This leaves out a lot of children with memory, visual processing, or other deficits. How far officials are willing to stretch the definition of learning disabled, in order to give students extra help in their area of weakness, depends on the state and the school system.

Since 1975, there has been a Public Law (94–142) mandating that all children receive free, appropriate public education regardless of the level or severity of their disability. This includes learning-disabled children, but, naturally, there have to be some criteria for determining which children need special help in the classroom. In 1986, a law was added, Public Law 99–457, that required the states to set aside money for the public school system to provide therapies and education for children aged three to five years who qualify as disabled in some category.

In general, I think the schools do an excellent job of accommodating so many different students with so many needs. No one who taught school before the 1970s can begin to understand all the duties and responsibilities now expected of teachers. However, the schools do not always have the tools, knowledge or time to find solutions to all the children's problems. Individual teachers may be understanding of a child's limitations or they may not be, depending on how rigid they are about how the material should be taught and about what measurements should be used to determine whether the child has learned it.

For example, Jeremy may perfectly understand the lessons he has learned about photosynthesis, but if he can't write well, he can't indicate on a test that he had understood the assigned chapter. If he can't read well, he can't understand the material unless it is presented orally. If he can't remember well, he needs more repetition or other strategies to help jog his memory.

Maria Menendez came to see us when she was in first grade, age seven. Despite her Hispanic names, she was second-generation American. Her parents had moved to the United States from Cuba as children when Castro came into power. She came from a long line of professionals, and her grandparents had done well in the United States, starting with a restaurant, and then, when their English improved, getting jobs with the Postal Service. Maria's parents were both lawyers. Making good grades was a given in their household.

Maria had talked early and could sing exactly on key even as a tiny girl. However, she had more difficulty learning to dress herself, to set the table and get the silverware in the right place, and to make the pretty tissue-paper flowers the preschool teacher showed them. She was left-handed and had difficulty using scissors. She had problems telling her left from her right. When she was in first grade, her mother still had to tie her shoes for her.

She was fascinated with nature and the outdoors. She could name every tree and flower and would often call them out when she and her father were taking walks together. The Discovery Channel was her favorite channel, and *Bambi* was her favorite movie, especially the part where Bambi and Thumper and Flower experience their first spring.

Maria enjoyed kindergarten, planting beans, playing with finger paints, singing songs. True, she had a little trouble when they did a dance for the parent–teacher association – she just couldn't seem to get the steps. But she sang so well that the teacher let her sing along with the tape, which made her feel like the star of the show.

"Mami, when I grow up I'm going to be a singer, a zookeeper, or a king," she told her mother.

"Not a queen?" asked her mother.

"No, kings have all the magnificence," she said.

Her mother laughed. Maria was always saying amusing things and entertaining everyone with her precocious vocabulary.

Maria started first grade with great excitement, but after several weeks, she seemed less enthusiastic.

"My teacher doesn't like me," she told her parents. "She says I need to try harder with my writing. She fusses at me when I write the arithmetic wrong."

Her parents reassured her that starting something new was always hard and that she would do fine. But a few weeks later, Maria came home, crying.

"Mami, Jessica says I'm stupid. She laughs at me when I read. And the teacher says that my papers look like chicken scratchings. I'm not stupid, am I, Mami? Why can't I write like the other children?"

The next day she came home with a 40 on an arithmetic paper. Maria had copied the problems down wrong from the board. She added the numbers together correctly, but they were the wrong problems. There was also a note from the teacher for the Menendezes to see her.

The teacher was brief. "Maria isn't going to pass first grade if she doesn't improve. She is working below grade level in math and writing, and she seems immature for her age. I think you should have her tested."

Maria's parents were stunned. Their bright and creative child was immature? The teacher was already warning that she would fail first grade about two months into the year? How could this be?

They agreed with the teacher that Maria needed testing to find out what was going on, although they didn't agree about what Maria's problems were. They came to us.

Maria's IQ was 111, in the high average range. However, she had strengths in certain subcategories of the test, such as verbal arithmetic, vocabulary, and analogies, and weaknesses in others, such as mazes and coding. There was a 20-point difference between the verbal and the performance portions of the test, which placed her in the superior range for verbal IQ and in the low average range for performance IQ. She blew the top off the receptive and expressive language testing. Her educational testing was generally average, but she got some of the arithmetic wrong because she didn't line up her numbers correctly. Though she clearly knew what she wanted to write, she reversed some of her letters and she pressed the pencil so deeply into the paper that she tore it at one point. She also kept her face right next to the paper and she held it sideways to write, a common left-handed behavior.

She had some mild difficulties with gross motor (big muscle) skills, such as skipping in a coordinated fashion, but she threw a ball well and could jump well from a height. In fine motor (small muscle) skills she had terrible trouble. She had difficulty building steps out of blocks. Her drawings were cramped and inaccurate. She couldn't button well. And she still didn't know her left from her right.

Further testing indicated that picking out patterns, finding pieces of a whole, and figuring out what was placed in her hand when her eyes were shut were all very difficult for her.

Maria was an intelligent and mature child with many gifts, but with a specific learning disability: she had visual motor and visual spatial problems. In other words, she had difficulty with anything involving moving her body in an pattern (such as dancing), had trouble figuring out where her body was in space if her eyes were closed, and had trouble transferring visual patterns, symbols, and shapes into something involving muscle use, such as a writing a word, doing a puzzle, or a tying a shoelace.

Maria clearly needed some modifications in the way that she was taught. She needed extra work in tracing letters, which she could practice in the sand, with finger paints, or on the mirror with shaving cream. An alphabet strip was placed on her desk to refer to in order to see whether her letters were in the right direction. She started learning to type on a keyboard and was allowed to record some of her work on a tape recorder to indicate her understanding of a subject. She did her arithmetic on graph paper so she could line the numbers up in the appropriate boxes. Flashcard drill helped her to distinguish between words like "saw" and "was." Smiling faces were drawn on the inside of her shoes so she could know which foot to put them on.

Maria and her mother enjoyed playing the games "Simon" and "Memory," both of which involve remembering patterns and where things are in space. She began karate to improve her balance and coordination.

With her parents and her teachers working with her and the knowledge of how to deal with her learning disability, Maria did well. Fortunately her school system was amenable to the changes in the way Maria learned. Not all school systems are so accommodating.

My strong opinion is that it doesn't matter how you learn as long as you're learning the material. In fact, a teacher who refuses to let a child do some of her work on a computer is actually keeping the child from learning some important skills for adult life. Once a child has mastered the concept behind long division, why in the world shouldn't she be allowed to do it on a calculator if she makes frequent mistakes in adding and subtracting? And if a student gives a presentation through artwork, drama, a PowerPoint presentation or orally instead of writing an essay, isn't he still integrating and explaining the material? However, some school administrators and teachers are very rigid. If the traditional method is good enough for the other kids, they think, why should they make an exception for one?

I feel it is important to find a happy medium. It is true that self-esteem and confidence are instilled best by meeting a challenge head on, struggling with it, and mastering it. Still, if a person is blind, he shouldn't be expected to walk around town without a cane or a seeing-eye dog. Success can be achieved in many ways. When Maria gets out of school, perhaps she will be a success as a musician, a business administrator, a journalist, a lawyer. She probably wouldn't be a good architect, sleight-of-hand magician or professional basketball player.

As I have learned over and over again, though, never say never about a child.

Chapter 11

Attention Deficit Hyperactivity Disorder and its Mimics

Tommy Bangs was the scapegrace of the school and the most trying little scapegrace that ever lived. As full of mischief as a monkey, yet so good-hearted that one could not help forgive his tricks, so scatter-brained that words went by him like the wind, yet so penitent for every misdeed, that it was impossible to keep sober when he vowed tremendous vows of reformation…Mr. and Mrs. Bhaer lived in a state of preparation for a mishap, from the breaking of Tommy's own neck, to the blowing up of the entire family with gun-powder, and Nursey had a particular drawer in which she kept bandages, plasters, and salves for his especial use…

If he did not know his lessons, he always had some droll excuse to offer, and as he was usually clever at his books, and as bright as a button at composing answers when he did not know them, he got on *pretty* well at school.

Louisa May Alcott, Little Men

There are days I wake up and don't want to go in to work. In fact, I don't even want to get out of bed! It would be so tempting to call in sick, but I think of the patients waiting for me. So I get myself out the door and begin my 30-minute drive to work along a country road. In the spring the redbuds and dogwoods are in bloom throughout the forest on either side of the road. I pass a creek which winds through pastureland with grazing cows and nursing calves. I see little colts next to their mothers, balancing on those frail legs that look as if they could barely hold the animals up. In the fall, the hardwood trees are red and gold, and the air is crisp, and the winter brings some days when icicles glisten on the branches of the trees.

I just about always see some animals along the way. There is a flock of wild turkeys in a small farming area called Cane Creek. Deer run across the road and groundhogs perch beside it, surveying the countryside in their shy way. There are hawks way up in the sky, with wings outstretched to catch the wind.

That morning drive is a time that I'm glad I live in the North Carolina countryside.

Then I get to work and, even if I'm tired, the children are waiting and very soon I find myself being pulled once more into this fascinating job of mine, with its non-stop activity.

The non-stop activity part is especially true when we have to evaluate a child with attention deficit hyperactivity disorder, or ADHD. I have to muster my energy from every possible source in order to keep up with them! Sometimes, after such a child leaves, our whole team is ready to take a nap and we wonder how in the world two parents manage when a whole crew of us end up exhausted after half a day.

One of my tricks is to take an exceptionally rambunctious child, put him in a chair with wheels, run him up and down the hall a few times and then slowly wheel him around. We look at the pictures on the walls, which are mostly of different animals or of children, and we talk about them. It always calms them down like a charm, though I don't know why. People who work with sensory motor integration would say it may be because I'm giving them the vestibular stimulation their bodies crave.

Some of the kids seem 100 percent obviously ADHD. They run into the waiting room, throw magazines on the floor, break something accidentally, dash in and out of the room, interrupt their parents, fidget incessantly, and turn immediately to a novel sound or visual stimulus ("What's that out in the hall?" "Did you hear that bird outside?" "How did that crack on the ceiling happen?"). They interrupt everything you say, become preoccupied with aspects of the tests that are unimportant, like the page numbers, and have to get up from the testing table many times. Sometimes children will even do their work standing up.

I'll never forget tiny Paula, the first and one of the very few three-year-olds I ever diagnosed with ADHD and medicated. We were expecting her and her mother at 2 p.m. At exactly 2, the door slammed, and a small, very cute pigtailed tornado came whirling into the office.

It said, "Hi – are you the doctor?" in a chipper voice, climbed on my lap, and began pulling all the drawers out of my desk.

"What is this? May I use it? May I have it? What is that picture? Uh-oh – I dropped it!"

Papers, paper clips, and pens were scattered all over the floor by this time.

"Mommy – hey, hey!" The tornado danced out of the office, pulling her mother by the hand as a woman came in the front door, looking very worried. "Come, come see! Toys!"

Then she crawled under the sofa. I knew what she had before I even began the interview process, looked at her ratings by questionnaire, or examined her. She also managed to pull out one of my earrings during the exam; luckily, it didn't tear my ear. There wasn't an aggressive or hateful bone in her body, though, and it was clear that she meant no harm. She was simply driven.

Whew!

To help show the complexity of this diagnosis, I include descriptions of some of the children who have been referred to us to rule out attention deficit disorder. See if it is evident which of the following kids truly has ADHD.

Anna is in kindergarten. She seems very shy and yet she hits and has temper tantrums when she does not get her way. She doesn't talk much, listen well, or stay in the group when they read a story or sing circle games; instead, she tends to wander around the room. Her favorite play area is the sand and water table, and she gets very restless when she's at the dress-up/housekeeping center where the other children play pretend games. Her parents say that she often leads them to what she wants instead of telling them to help her.

Tommy is two-and-a-half. He has been very active since he learned to walk. His mother can't take her eyes off him for 30 seconds without his getting into mischief. He wants to do everything his older brothers do and often manages to keep up with them. The day before his visit to the DEC, he flushed the metal roll on the toilet-paper holder down the toilet and emptied the toothpaste tube on the floor while his mother was answering the phone.

Roberto is six. He is an only child and when he was a baby, he was quite ill. His parents have always worried he would get sick again and are extra gentle with him. Still, he is a healthy and stocky boy who is big for his age. He is very difficult to manage in school: won't listen, is aggressive to the other children, refuses to do his share of clean-up, runs off from the lunch line. He is reasonably good at his work when the teachers can get him to do it. His mother has the same problems at home and always has had. At the office, when he runs off she says, "Roberto, would you like to come back and see the lady?" When he hits, she says, "That's not nice, Roberto," but makes no effort to stop him.

Michael is seven. His mother is a single parent. His father has little contact with the family and has a lot of difficulty keeping a job. His mother seems to make a strong effort to be consistent in disciplining him, but it has always been a challenge and he has always been very active, almost "like the Energizer bunny; he keeps going and going." Michael had some speech therapy in preschool but seems to have no speech problems now. At school he can't focus well, he fidgets and interrupts the teacher frequently. Sometimes he seems sleepy and yawns a lot, but his mother says he gets plenty of sleep. When the teacher sits right beside him and gives him constant encouragement, he can get his work done and does a good job.

Carla is six. She lives in a house with her mother, the mother's boyfriend, and a little brother. She did not seem exceptionally active or distractible when she was younger; this behavior began about a year ago. At this time she also began being moody, hypersensitive (crying easily), and very hostile to her mother. She tells the psychologist at the office that "I do bad things and don't listen because Boogie makes me." She cannot answer the question, "Who is Boogie?" In a family picture, she draws herself small on the very edge of the page and draws her mother's boyfriend very large and on the other side of the paper.

As you may have guessed, Michael is the one with true ADHD (and his father probably has it, too). This may seem self-evident but, in these cases, all the children were referred to us for the same reported problems: distractibility, poor attention, high activity level, and behavior problems.

The others might have ADHD, but it is much more likely that Anna has a language disorder, Tommy is just an active two-year-old with good motor skills, Roberto has been given inconsistent discipline, and Carla may be suffering from post-traumatic stress disorder caused by sexual abuse.

There is an enormous amount of controversy about the diagnosis and treatment of attention deficit hyperactivity disorder. Although I assume most of the readers of this book are familiar with the term and its symptoms, I will give a fairly brief description of the characteristics of ADHD. It consists of two major symptoms, hyperactivity-impulsivity and inattention. The kids who have the hyperactive behaviors along with the inattention are much easier to pick out. There is a subtype of children who only have the inattention, which is called attention deficit disorder (ADD) or, more confusingly, ADHD without hyperactivity.

The symptoms of ADHD have to occur in more than one setting and they have to have been present for at least six months; I would say usually, longer. Sometimes a child will start having symptoms when he or she enters kindergarten because the need for concentration is so much greater than what they experienced in their environment before. More boys have ADHD than girls, but it can be noticed in both.

Hyperactive-impulsive children are squirmy in the seat and often in and out of the seat. They seem to be driven by a motor, going on and on, running, climbing, jumping. They don't seem to have much sense of danger. For example, the child may ride his bike down a hill and crash and even though hurt, go right back and do it again. Parents often report that it is hard to take them out to the mall or a restaurant because they run away or are unintentionally disruptive to other people. They often talk non-stop and blurt out answers at school. Even if made to raise their hands, they are the kids who raise their hand and wave wildly in the air, yelling, "I know, teacher, I know. Pick me!" They can be quite unpopular with other children because they leap before they look and have trouble following the rules of a game, have trouble waiting in line, have trouble keeping their hands to themselves, and often get the whole class in trouble.

A child who acts this way is not "just mean," as they say here in the South. They are often generous and loving. They just can't seem to control themselves.

Most children who are hyperactive are also inattentive. Children who have ADD alone are often thought to be "slow," easily getting confused, doing poorly in school, and never quite seeming to be "with the class." These children are easily distracted by the person walking outside the classroom, by the crack in their desktop, or the hum of the air conditioner. They forget their books, their homework, or that their father told them to take out the garbage. Their rooms and desks are disaster zones. They have trouble finishing a task or activity. When all the other children have finished their reading, they are still staring into space, "wool gathering." They notice little details that are not relevant. I will be talking to a child and ask him a question and he will point and say, "Does that bag have your lunch in it?"

The diagnosis is relatively common and it is not unusual for me to be asked to observe a child in a classroom for ADHD and to say to the teacher afterwards, "Well, Carlos doesn't look so bad, but that child over there…does *he* ever need to be seen!" Incidentally, when I, as the new visitor, enter the classroom, all the children are interested and distracted by my presence. It is the child with ADHD who keeps staring back at me and trying to engage in conversation fifteen minutes later when the others have forgotten all about me.

It is my strong opinion that ADHD is a real diagnosis, but so many other problems mimic it and display similar symptoms that, unless the child is evaluated very thoroughly, a misdiagnosis can easily be made. A child who has some of the above problems may not actually have ADHD. The child may be depressed or developmentally delayed; have an anxiety disorder, a chronic illness, a learning disability, bipolar illness; or is just very active but attends well. In a standard doctor office visit, it is very hard to tease all these factors out. And frequently the parents and teachers are pushing the doctor for a quick solution to the problem.

Therefore, it is very important to eliminate these possibilities before placing a child on stimulant medication. Might a child with one of these other diagnoses also have ADHD? Absolutely. But there is no way to determine that without treating the initial problem first.

The most common argument I hear about the diagnosis of ADHD being a myth is that there is no blood test or other test that can confirm the diagnosis. This is true. However, it is also true about many other medical and psychiatric conditions such as depression, schizophrenia, obsessive compulsive disorder, autism, Tourette syndrome, irritable bowel syndrome, chronic fatigue syndrome, fibromyalgia, and many others. I have never heard anyone say that schizophrenia is not a true diagnosis because there is no blood test for it. These diagnoses and many others are based on two things: careful delineation and observation of behavior based on a previous set of standards, and elimination of other problems that might mimic the condition.

Furthermore, anyone who has seen the father of a child with ADHD fidget, pace the floor, and interrupt knows that there is a genetic component to this problem. In fact, it's not unusual to have a father come up later after his child has been diagnosed with ADHD and say, "You know, I always thought I was just stupid or something, but now I am pretty sure that I have this problem, too."

The other argument I hear against the treatment of ADHD is that the medicines commonly used to treat it have many side effects. Actually, Ritalin, Adderal and related drugs have far fewer side effects than many other medications, especially if given in appropriate doses. The most common side effects are loss of appetite, headaches, stomach-aches, moodiness when the medication wears off, and what I call the "he's-just-not-the-same-child-any-more" side effect, which I don't fully understand but have seen. Most of these are dose-related or time-related and can be eliminated. If they can't be eliminated, the medication can be stopped, and all of these medications are out of one's system by the end of the day. There is also a new medicine, Stratera, which has even fewer side effects.

I do think that the number of children treated for this condition is appalling, especially in the United States. This is partly related to misdiagnosis, as I have explained. However, it is my personal, unproven theory that, just as there is a critical time for the brain to master language, music, and math, there is probably a critical time for learning to pay attention and focus. When we compare the activities in which small children engaged, say, in the mid-1970s to the activities they engage in now, there is far less opportunity today for children to learn the skills needed to focus and pay attention.

When I was very small and acted bored, I remember my mother handing me the box in which she kept her buttons. I spent a long time sorting them by color, sorting them by size, picking out the prettiest ones, and arranging them in patterns. I spent time listening to story records and drawing or looking at books while I listened. I played outside in the woods or with the neighborhood children. I rarely watched television. By the time I started school, I had a lot of experience with sustained, self-motivated attention.

Furthermore, in preschool and kindergarten, I painted with finger paints, participated in pageants and plays, played singing and dancing games, ran outside, planted beans in plastic cups, and pretended. I was not required to do worksheets circling the picture that begins with "b" or to read (which a vast number of kindergartens require by the end of the year now). I learned to pay attention through more movement and hands-on tasks. Although I learned to focus and concentrate on age-appropriate things, less difficult and tedious material was required of me at a young age. Because I enjoyed and was not overwhelmed with the work, I did not show fidgetiness and inattention. Nevertheless, I very quickly learned to read in first grade when the concepts were presented to me.

I am not referring to the child who learns to read on his or her own at an early age. I am talking more about children who are not developmentally ready to read who are pressured to do so and become avoidant of school-work and who feel stupid. They may look as if they have ADHD when, in fact, they are just feeling overwhelmed. Most of us would probably fidget, daydream a lot, and feel like an idiot in a nuclear physics class.

Most early elementary classes are geared to children (read: "girls") who are able to express their thoughts and feelings verbally, cooperate and not aggressively compete, and who can sit still for a lengthy period of time. The child who prefers to learn in physical ways is not often the teacher's pet.

I have seen a range of children with ADHD. I recommend behavior and environmental modifications for all of them and medicine for many. Medicine does have some fantastic results for many children, which makes them, their parents, and their teachers much happier. I have never seen a child become addicted to the medicine, but I have certainly seen many children who want to take it because they know that it will make it so much easier for them to succeed in life and get along with others.

Chapter 12

Up and Down: Mood Disorders

He rolls onto his stomach, pulling the pillow tight around his head, blocking out the sharp arrows of sun that pierce through the window. Morning is not a good time for him. Too many details crowd his mind. Brush his teeth first? Wash his face? What pants should he wear? What shirt? The small seed of despair cracks open and sends experimental tendrils upward to the fragile skin of calm holding him together. Are You On the Right Road?

Crawford had tried to prepare him for this. "It's all right Con, to feel anxious. Allow yourself a couple of bad days, now and then, will you?"

Sure. How bad? Razor-blade bad? He had wanted to ask, but he hadn't...

Judith Guest, Ordinary People

When I was in my residency, I admitted a girl who had taken an overdose of aspirin and Tylenol. Tylenol is actually an extremely dangerous medication to take in overdose since it causes serious harm to the liver. Fortunately she had been discovered shortly after she had taken the medicine and we were able to get it out of her system. This included putting a tube down to her stomach and pulling the contents up with a syringe, having her drink horrible activated charcoal milkshakes (very thick and black), and take an even more disgusting medication called Mucomist.

She was a very attractive 16-year-old girl with thick dark hair, a heart-shaped face, and dark hazel eyes. Apparently, her family had moved from Saudi Arabia several years previously. She spoke accented but fluent

English. Her father and brother came to see her in the hospital and shortly we heard crying and a lot of harsh, angry Arabic in male voices directed at Yasmin, our patient. The nurses came in to see what was going on. They came in just as the father was slapping the girl across the face. She was sobbing. The nurses restored order and escorted the father and brother out, with him still yelling at her over his shoulder.

We could not get Yasmin to talk for a few days except to cry and say, "I don't want to go home" and "I wish I were dead." She did have some whispered conversations on the phone with someone but she always hung up the minute someone came in. She was supervised carefully during her recovery to make sure she did not attempt to kill herself again. When she was well enough, she was transferred to the psychiatric unit for severe depression with suicidal intent.

The day before she left for the psychiatric ward, Yasmin confided in me about what was going on. Her parents meant well, she said, but they were very distrustful of Americans and American culture. They didn't allow her to make any friends at all and she was told that she must not talk to anyone at school. Her brother would come home and tell on her if he saw her being friendly with someone. She was to come home immediately after school and was not allowed outside of the house. She could not talk on the phone. She could not read American novels, only textbooks. She was required to wait on her father and brother, as was her mother, hand and foot.

Her brother, a year older, was allowed complete freedom to come and go as he wished. Her father had begun making her receive visits, fully chaperoned, from a Saudi man in his late twenties whose parents were friends of her parents. She knew that an arranged marriage was eventually intended, but she was frightened of the man.

"If we were still living in Saudi Arabia," she said, "I would still be kept away from boys and kept mainly in the house. But I would have girlfriends to visit with and gossip with. I did before. We would dance together and do our homework in groups. Also, my family would have friends over and I would be allowed to visit with the other family. Here, I have no one. I am so lonely. America is different and it's not as dangerous or bad as my father thinks."

Tears rolled down her face again. "I try to talk to him about this, but all he does is yell and hit me," she said.

I asked about the phone calls. Yasmin colored and became silent for a while.

"I have a friend," she whispered. "A boy. We met at school. He's very nice and he would never hurt me or make me want to do anything I didn't want to do. I'm a chaste girl," she insisted. "I wouldn't do something bad."

"Is that who you were talking to on the phone?" I asked.

"Yes. Him and his mother," she admitted, looking down. "He has taken me to visit his mother after school. My family doesn't know. They think I am taking the bus home right after school, but sometimes they drive me home after a visit and let me off a block away. My brother doesn't know because he plays basketball after school. He gets to do *everything* he wants," she said resentfully.

"Darlene – that's my friend Robert's mother – says that I can come live with them if I want," she told me. "I would love to. But my family would kill me if they found out that I was visiting them. I have to keep my whole life a secret."

I was really alarmed by this whole story and terribly sympathetic with her plight. However, if her parents weren't starving her, weren't beating her to leave bruises, were providing a home for her and were living by their cultural expectations, could it be determined that this was abuse?

The day she went to the psychiatric ward, I called the Arabic League, which gave me the name of a Saudi psychologist who often served as a cultural liaison to Arabic families who lived in the Minneapolis area. I told her the situation. She sighed deeply.

"Yes, this is not that uncommon," she said. "I actually know this family. We have had dealings with them before because the father's boss was upset by the way he treated the female workers in the restaurant. It is very difficult when two so very different cultures clash. I will talk to them and do my best."

In the meantime, I became busy with other patients who came newly to our service, but my medical students and I tried to visit Yasmin every day that we could. She did seem to be better, but nothing had really changed with her situation except that she now had to deal with a number of emotionally troubled teens on the ward. Darlene and Robert called regularly but were not allowed to talk to her. Her father visited her only now and then and the visits were acrimonious. I saw her mother once, a small, dark shadow behind her husband, her face covered with a veil. Yasmin also got in trouble with the ward nurses for trying to sneak to the telephone in the night and make a call.

I was allowed to read her chart. There were copious notes about her manipulative behavior, trying to wheedle privileges out of the nurses, using her relationship with me to try to get me to intervene for her, trying to turn Darlene and Robert against her parents. I was furious. What other options did she have? However, the psychiatry ward saw it differently.

The Saudi psychologist spoke to me again. She had tried very hard to reason with the parents, she said, but they would not listen. The father was determined to live as much as possible as if they were still in Saudi Arabia. He had come to the United States for better job opportunities but he was horrified by everything about the country's culture. He was determined the "devils" would not pollute his daughter. He felt that everything he was doing was in her best interest.

Yasmin was eventually able to convince the hospital doctors that she was no longer suicidal. I came to visit her one day and discovered that she had been discharged back to her home. I tried to call her home, but no one would answer the phone. I didn't know what to do. Darlene called me, having been given my number by Yasmin. She was crying on the phone and saying, "I love that little girl. I want so badly to help her." I didn't know what to tell her.

Three weeks later, Yasmin came into the hospital in a coma. She had taken an overdose of her antidepressant medication and this time she could not be revived. Her parents wept and raged and said it was all the fault of the evil country in which they lived. My resentment against the family and the psychiatric ward boiled within me but I could do nothing.

I tell this story partly because it still sometimes wakes me in the night, and partly to bring up a number of points. First, just because a person is depressed because of their circumstances doesn't mean that they aren't truly clinically depressed. So many times depression is brushed off because, "well, who wouldn't be depressed if that had happened to them?"

Second, this story is a warning that sometimes people who are severely depressed have too little energy to kill themselves. Then, when they get a little better, they appear more cheerful because they have the energy to commit suicide and they feel they have a way out of their misery. Full bottles of antidepressants and other drugs should be kept far out of reach of a person who has been suicidal.

And third, the gulfs between cultures can be as wide as the Grand Canyon, and as deep. I felt, and still feel, that this family was abusing this girl but they obviously felt that they were protecting her from bad influences. I have no answer for this problem. I do know that sometimes my colleagues and I can't get through to a family or change patterns that we feel are bad for a child because of cultural differences, even those that are smaller, such as the differences between black, Hispanic, and white America.

We now know that people of any age, including infants, can be depressed. We took care of a nine-month-old whose mother died, who lost developmental milestones and became lethargic until she came out of foster care and was given to her maternal aunt. She then gained back the skills she had lost and developed normally.

Children often demonstrate depression by showing irritability and acting out. By far the most dramatic case of this I have ever seen was a child named Amy. She was a six-year-old who was removed from her mother for neglect and placed with her father and stepmother. The father and his new wife had two boys and a little girl together who were among the sweetest, most thoughtful, and most polite children I have ever met. Amy was only one year older than the oldest boy.

The biological mother was also a nice woman, but a combination of stress, financial problems, and a bad choice of boyfriends had led to her providing inadequate care for Amy.

Amy's father and his new family were very ready to welcome Amy into the fold. However, even the best intended and most stable of families can begin to fall apart under tremendous stress. Amy was absolutely impossible to manage. She was wildly active, destructive with toys, aggressive to her new siblings, and very distractible. She seemed to particularly misbehave around her stepmother, who was trying very hard to manage four children and attend part-time night college at the same time. It soon became clear she would need to quit her schooling for a while and concentrate on Amy.

Amy was so difficult and wild and the situation so desperate that, despite my common choice not to treat children for ADHD until their other problems are dealt with, I did put Amy on Ritalin. Things seemed better very briefly and then got much worse. Amy began urinating on clean laundry and in her closet and smearing feces on the wall. She tore holes in the carpet and the curtains. Her tantrums were uncontrollable. She called her stepmother horrible names.

"Stupid bitch," she'd yell, in front of the other children. "I hate you. You're a shitty poophead."

We stopped the Ritalin with no improvement. I arranged for counseling, but we could not get an appointment for her for several months.

I became convinced that Amy was seriously emotionally disturbed, possibly even psychotic, and arranged for her to be admitted to a psychiatric hospital on an emergency basis. The parents were willing at that point because they were truly at the end of their rope and Amy's behavior was causing the other children to show emotional problems.

Furthermore, the stepmother would not have been human if she had not begun to feel resentful of the child and have trouble treating her with the love with which she treated her own. After all, she was the main caretaker of a difficult child who was not even related to her.

The psychiatric hospital, which shall remain nameless, took Amy off the Ritalin and put her on Dexedrine, a related substance. Amy remained in the hospital for three or four days and behaved fairly well in the new setting. Therefore the psychiatrist concluded that the problem lay entirely with the parents and discharged her.

The poor parents didn't know what to do. They begged the psychiatrist to further evaluate and treat Amy before sending her back home. They told him they had no idea how they were going to manage having Amy back without a major change in her behavior.

The psychiatrist threw up his hands.

"All right," he said. "Fine. We'll keep her and I'll charge you with abandonment of your child."

They took Amy back home. For the first time, Amy began to cry in grief, not in fury.

"I want to go back to my Mama," she said over and over. "I want my Mama."

By then Amy's mother had moved out of her boyfriend's house, had a job, and was keeping the house in better condition. It was arranged through social services for Amy to return to her mother's care, at least on a temporary basis. Amy was also able to get an appointment with a counselor.

As soon as Amy returned home, her behavior improved markedly. She began to smile and laugh more. She covered her mother with hugs and kisses. It was as if she were a different child. She had been severely depressed because of the separation from her mother.

The biological mother, understandably, I suppose, blamed her behavior on the father and stepmother, but I am convinced that they went far, far, beyond the call of duty in trying to raise Amy. This was not their fault – it was the fault of childhood depression. They have Amy over some weekends and she does relatively well now that she knows she will be going home to her beloved mother.

Another mood disorder that is very hard to diagnose correctly in children is bipolar illness (also called manic-depressive illness). In fact, though I have read a good bit about it and been to several conferences on bipolar illness, I always feel more comfortable if I get a second opinion from a child psychiatrist. I suspect it when there is a child who has a diagnosis of ADHD who, if anything, seems to get worse on stimulant medication. They are often aggressive, have extreme outbursts (similar to Amy), and are very, very impulsive, often doing things that are "crazy" more than the impulsiveness of a child with standard ADHD that might manifest itself in such things as answering a question before it is asked. An elementary-school child who is doing things like starting the family car and going for a joyride in the middle of the night may have more going on.

Doug Mahoney was a child I saw for follow-up for years. He was initially referred in second grade because of ADHD symptoms and poor school performance. His life was fraught with problems and his diagnosis was complicated. His mother died when he was four and his grandfather and father were raising him. The grandfather had many health problems and also drank to excess at times. The father was a used car dealer and was often gone for lengthy periods of time. In fact, although I spoke to him on the phone, I didn't meet his father for many years after I began seeing Doug.

His grandfather did the best he could, considering the circumstances, but Doug was always exceptionally difficult and strong-willed and the grandfather would throw up his hands and say he couldn't control him. They frequently had yelling matches that were heard all through the neighborhood. The neighbors had called Social Services several times but the case was closed each time for lack of evidence of true neglect or abuse. The family was just "sorry," as they would say in this area.

I did feel Doug had ADHD and stimulant medication did seem to benefit him some. His fourth-grade teacher took special interest in him and often took him places after school or had him to her house on the weekend as a reward for good behavior. That year he behaved quite well. He was put in a special reading class, which improved his school performance a little.

However, whenever he would come to see me for follow-up – always with his grandfather – they would jaw back and forth. Mr. Mahoney would tell me how impossible Doug was: he wouldn't do any chores, he was disrespectful, he didn't come home in time for dinner, and he kept everything a mess. I urged behavioral and family counseling but they were a country family to whom that was extremely foreign and distasteful. Still, Doug did better with teachers he liked and he could be quite cooperative and endearing.

Doug's behavior deteriorated more in middle school and he grew quite strong and tall so that his grandfather was almost scared to discipline him. His grades slipped and he began refusing to take his medicine, although his teachers said they could tell a difference when he did take it.

"I don't have to put up with this from you," his grandfather would yell. "One of these days I'll leave you high and dry."

"You just do that," Doug would yell back. "I can take care of myself a whole lot better without you."

"The hell you can," Mr. Mahoney would say. "You'd last two days, tops. You're worthless. You're going to end up in the High Rise [the juvenile detention center] and then you'll be sorry you treated me so bad."

And so on.

It was in high school that Doug's life really began to come apart. First of all, he had never been academically capable and the work was very difficult for him, even through he was in some of the slower track classes. Many of the kids were from different schools and made fun of his "redneck" ways. He developed intense prejudice against the Mexican and Asian kids in the school and made very inappropriate remarks. The girls complained that he said obscene or frightening things to them. He was put into in-school suspension numerous times.

I had many conversations with Mr. Mahoney on the phone and met with Doug. Doug began being very hostile to me, too. No longer could Mr. Mahoney's usual remedy for Doug's behavior, "I want you to talk to the boy, Dr. Hays, and set him straight," work. He seemed very depressed but refused to take any medicine or talk to a professional. Everything was someone else's fault.

Doug got suspended for four days for getting into a fight with a senior who was a football player. Though it was clear that he would get slaughtered, he was the one who had provoked the fight. The school had a meeting that included the guidance counselor, the principal, his homeroom teacher, the school patrol officer, Mr. Mahoney, and me. His father could not be there.

"Doug, you have got to get control of yourself," said the principal. "You've made a lot of kids so angry that they're out to get you. The Mexican gang has it in for you. It's really unsafe for you to be here if you continue to act the way you do."

"The hell with you. You're not the boss of me," Doug snapped. "I'm better than any of them. Those asshole Tacos ain't worth shit. I'm going to beat up the whole gang of them."

"*Doug!* You cannot talk like that here!" Everyone had recoiled in horror at his words.

"I don't care how I talk." Doug raised his voice. "I'm going to get me an 18-wheeler, steal me some money, and drive off to California. That's the last I'll see of you shitheads."

Mr. Mahoney grabbed his arm roughly. Doug shook him off.

"Doug, you're failing your classes," said the guidance teacher. "You never turn in any homework. You're not even trying."

"I'm smarter than anyone in this school," said Doug. "No one is going to tell me what to do, ever. I'm going to get me a job and make millions of dollars and buy up this school and get it torn down."

It was obvious Doug could not be reasoned with. It was also obvious that he was severely troubled. He refused to see a psychologist or go to the hospital and he was strong enough that he would have to be fought down and dragged by several people if he were to go. The school patrol officer was alerted to keep an eye on Doug when he returned and I planned to call a lawyer to find out what could be legally done to get Doug professional help.

One of the things that made me think that Doug might well have bipolar illness was his pattern of depression and wild behavior that included "grandiose" statements. Grandiose means beliefs that one is all-powerful, untouchable, capable beyond any reality. Doug's comments seemed to me to be more than the useless threats of a trapped teenager.

Doug finished his suspension the next day and was allowed back at school. By 11 a.m. on a busy day with patients I got another panicked call from Mr. Mahoney.

"Do something!" he said. "The school just called. Doug is telling everyone he's got a gun at home and that he's going to come and shoot everyone in the school. They're taking him to the police station."

"I knew this was going to happen sometime," he told me. "He's just no good through and through."

I explained to Mr. Mahoney that I thought Doug had a mental illness and needed hospitalization and medication. As soon as I could, I talked to the guidance counselor and to Social Services.

Doug was taken to the juvenile detention center instead of to a psychiatrist. I talked to the doctors there. Things were out of my hands but they did listen to me. They arranged for a psychiatrist to see him. Unfortunately Doug provoked a fight with several boys in the meantime and got beaten up. He got to the psychiatrist's office with two black eyes and a broken arm, still kicking and yelling.

The psychiatrist also felt that Doug was bipolar and began him on medication. Doug was sent for the rest of the school year, and possibly longer, to an organization that worked with troubled youth in an outdoor, rough-it setting. Mr. Mahoney moved elsewhere without leaving an address and I have to confess that I have lost touch with Doug and his family.

I hope he is doing better. I think he is potentially salvageable but only with medication, therapy, and, I hope, with the strict but caring discipline that can be provided where he is. What is to be done with all the Dougs of the world who don't get the help they need? Quite possibly, they will end up in prison for wild and purposeless crimes, or dead, or even, as in Doug's case, with a gun at school, shooting people randomly. Society must not abandon or ignore these children. And as we have learned to our detriment in such places as Columbine or Santee, we must jump to attention and alert the appropriate people when these children give out a cry for help.

Chapter 13

Cerebral Palsy

Walking, walking, walking, walking,
Seems so easy now!
But I remember when I was small
And I did not know how.
I would take two steps
And then four more
And bump my bottom on the floor!
Dad would say,
"That's okay –
Try again some other day."

Hap Palmer and Martha Cheney © 1983 Hap-Pal Music from
the CD Peek-A-Boo and video, Babysongs (www.happalmer.com)

The children with cerebral palsy who come to the office for speech or
physical therapy on a regular basis always light up our day. Whether they
crawl down the hall, flopping their bodies around, or walk on their tiptoes,
leaning precariously forward as if they might fall any minute, or weave from
side to side, or push themselves laboriously forward with a walker, or
proudly and ecstatically walk for the first time, they are almost always
striving to make new physical gains and are delighted to show off their
newfound skills. Their efforts to acquire new skills are a lesson in determination.

When I used to do hospital work and sometimes had to hurt children to
draw their blood or do other procedures, a kindly grandmother would

invariably say to me, "Oh, I could never do your job. I'm much too tenderhearted."

I never particularly looked on this as a compliment.

"Yes," I was always tempted to say, "I really enjoy inflicting pain upon little kids. That's why I love my work."

Similarly, I don't think parents of children with cerebral palsy or other disabilities particularly appreciate it when others say, "Oh, I can't imagine how you manage. You're so brave. You've been so patient."

I think what they would like to respond is, "Hey, I didn't ask to be elected to this position. However, having been given this task as part of my life, I have risen to the challenge and have come to discover the special rewards and the joys that it brings. That doesn't mean it's not hard, and sometimes I wish I weren't doing it. But it is my job and I'm dedicated to it."

The children have never known anything different but, if they were asked, I suspect they, too, would say that they're determined to make the best of a situation they didn't ask for.

Cerebral palsy is one of those terms like "developmental delay" that can mean a wide variety of conditions. Put quite simply, it means that the motor (muscle control) area of the brain is not working properly. Although, as many people think, it can be caused by lack of oxygen during the delivery, this is by no means the only way that it occurs. Most frequently, we do not know why a child has cerebral palsy. Sometimes it is because of something that happened while the baby was growing in the womb. Sometimes it is hereditary. It may be a stroke. Sometimes it is a premature birth.

It can affect the muscles by making them too spastic (tight and hyper-reactive), too hypotonic (loose and poorly reactive to sensation), or poorly coordinated. There can be problems with keeping the muscles still, which causes constant bobbing, jerking, or shaking, and there can be problems with balance. And all of these problems can be either mild or severe.

Athetoid cerebral palsy (difficulty controlling involuntary movements) used to be more common when we did not know how to treat jaundice with phototherapy, letting ultraviolet light break up the chemicals that can eventually build up and harm some of the balance pathways of the brain.

However, the damage that results from intraventricular hemorrhages that can occur in premature infants has caused some babies to have spastic cerebral palsy. As children survive at earlier and earlier gestational ages, now even at 23 weeks' gestation (very little more than half a pregnancy), they can have more chronic complications. When I was working in neonatal intensive care units in the 1980s, we rarely had a child younger than 26 or 27 weeks survive, whereas now we see a few of the children born at 23 weeks' gestation who are perfectly normal. It boggles the mind. Although I am generally pro-choice, I have gradually come to oppose third trimester abortions as we learn more about fetal development and improve our neonatal skills. By that time these fetuses have brain waves that mimic those of a newborn. How can we justify aborting babies who could survive outside the womb?

People criticize doctors for "playing God," but modern medicine has developed to the point where sometimes it isn't clear whether "playing God" means letting a child die or letting a child live. Decisions like these are fraught with moral complications.

I saw a little girl, Sasha, who was ten months old and born about two-and-a-half months premature. She was already considerably behind in some of her motor skills, more than would be accounted for by the complications from her prematurity. She had difficulty sucking and controlling her saliva so she drooled and bubbled, requiring suction. She had to be fed mainly by a tube going directly into her stomach because food and liquid would often go down the wrong way. Her legs were stiff and though she was learning to sit, she fell to the side often because she had not learned to protect and stabilize herself with her hands.

I tested Sasha's gross motor skills and they were at about the five-month level. Her language skills were also behind because of her severe problems with controlling the muscles of her mouth. However, her receptive language skills, such as turning to her name, understanding "no," looking directly up at a sound, and playing pat-a-cake and knowing bye-bye were normal. Also her mother indicated that she used two signs: "mama" and "drink." Her fine motor skills, the way she used her hands, were normal. Her cognitive skills were normal.

When I took out the stethoscope to start to examine her, this ten-month-old infant absolutely floored me. She looked right at me and put her hands up to her ears. She knew what I did with the stethoscope and she was showing me that I was going to put the ends in my ears!

A magnetic resonance image (MRI) showed that Sasha had had a stroke in fetal life. We don't know why. Like other children I had seen, Sasha was "locked in" – able to understand much more than her cerebral palsy allowed her to demonstrate. Nevertheless, she was doing a pretty good job. I have high hopes for her learning in the future and perhaps, as her brain grows, other neurons will take over some of the function of the damaged tissue.

Cerebral palsy does not get worse; if it does, some other neurologic condition is causing the symptoms that led to the muscle damage. For example, we currently see a child whose worsening ability to balance was found to be related to a metabolic disease. Now that it is being treated with special supplements, the damage has slowed.

Treatments continue to advance for these "locked in" children with celebral palsy. There is now augmentative communication, ways for children who cannot speak well to communicate. This includes computers that let children press certain buttons which actually vocalize what they are trying to say, for example, "Please get me the book" or "I need to go to the bathroom." Picture boards with signs to indicate certain needs are also used.

Small amounts of botulinum toxin, called Botox,[12] can be injected into tight muscles to stop spasticity, at least temporarily. For a child who has more widespread spasticity, a pump with a muscle relaxer can actually be implanted for a steady flow of medication onto the nerve roots. There is transelectrical stimulation, originally developed for astronauts, which may be able to passively increase muscle bulk in children who have flaccid muscles.[13] This treatment's efficacy is still in question. There is the common "release" of muscles that have stiffened to the point of being stuck by making a "z" cut in the tendon to lengthen it. There is also dorsal rhizotomy,[14] still a difficult choice for parents to make for their children, because it is major surgery that requires an enormous amount of follow-up therapy. First, the doctor electrically stimulates the nerves in the spinal cord, to figure out which ones are malfunctioning. Then the doctor teases out the problem nerve rootlets emerging from the spinal cord and cuts some of them. The previously spastic child can be left weak and flaccid and then has to work to gain back strength. However, I have seen videos of the end results and they can be very impressive.

With all these dramatic interventions, I'm still a big believer in speech, occupational, and physical therapy. Today there is a trend towards general family support and overall stimulation through play instead of these specialized therapies. But they can still work extremely well, assuming they are not the old-fashioned kind of therapy, where the parent is left out in the waiting room while the therapist performs some sort of "mysterious treatment," eventually bringing the child back to the parent. Instead, the parent needs to be involved every step of the way and shown how to work with the child at home.

Lela, the physical therapist, and I laugh that the room where we evaluate the children's motor skills is a "magic room" because it is amazing how often a child does something for the first time while being evaluated. First steps are taken, children pull up on furniture, or even jump. There are a lot of parental tears of joy shed in that room. I think the magic is related to showing children how a skill can be achieved and then letting their natural desire to move do the rest.

Gabriel, a child with cerebral palsy that we had been seeing for treatment for a full year, came in walking for the first time. As it was near Easter, Wilson invited him to come into his office to get some candy. Gabriel and his father slowly made their way down the hall, the boy stopping to look at every picture on the wall as he went and then tottering forward. When he reached the office, Wilson, the educational diagnostician, asked, "Do you want some chocolate?"

Gabriel grinned delightedly and, still standing, began bouncing and twisting, shaking his limbs to his own private music. Wilson watched in amusement and surprise.

"It's always this way," said his father, laughing. "He dances for chocolate. Say the word and the next thing you know, he's Elvis!"

Everyone is stimulated by joy to move and, given my love for chocolate, I might dance, too, if that were the best way to get it. But what really makes me want to dance for joy sometimes is the progress children can make when they are getting the right kind of help and encouragement.

Chapter 14

Autistic Spectrum Disorders

> If a man does not keep pace with his companions,
> perhaps it is because he hears a different drummer.
> Let him step to the music which he hears, however
> measured or far away.
>
> *Henry David Thoreau, Walden*

"The child you're seeing today sure is a cutie-pie," said Pam, our reception-ist. "Big brown eyes and little pigtails. Her mama's got her dressed like a little doll!"

"Let's see her picture," I said. We always take a picture of each child with our digital camera, decorate the edges with some interesting frame (comput-ers make artists of us all), put one copy in the chart, and give one to the family. It helps us to remember the child, and the parents are delighted. They often ask for several copies or pictures of other children who are with them.

"I'm waiting to get one later," said Pam. "She wouldn't look at the camera or smile this morning. Maybe she just got up too early."

"Yeah, maybe," I said. "I hope that's all."

Holly was referred at age four by a kind and beloved community doctor of the old school, who tended to protect parents from possible bad news and was quick to tell them that "she will outgrow it." Holly's parents were older and had had little previous experience with young children, so that it was difficult for them to know what behavior was age-appropriate and what was unusual. However, they had been having some concerns about Holly for a while. Though affectionate and cheerful, Holly did not talk, at least not any language that was intelligible. She did make strings of sounds with conversation-like intonation and she did use a few of her own made-up words. For example, "noob" meant she wanted a drink, though her family had no idea why.

Sometimes, to their surprise, she would say a word and then never say it again. When they went to the local spring festival, Holly pointed at a performing band and said, "saxophone," and it was beautifully articulated.

Holly loved her stuffed animals, and her extended family had provided for her generously. She had about 50 animals, from standard teddy bears to an armadillo that her aunt had brought back from Texas. She spent hours lining them up in a parade and then marching back and forth along the line like a field general commanding the troops. The animals were always put in exactly the same order. If someone tried to move one, or if one got misplaced and couldn't be put in its place, Holly would become inconsolable. She would cry and squeal and walk around the house, searching everywhere frantically until she found it. When she lost her pink elephant at the park, her father had to go out at night to Toys "R" Us and buy her an identical one so the family could get some sleep. When her father brought it home, she sniffed it and was not happy until her mother ran it in the dryer with fabric conditioner so that it would smell the same as it had before.

She also loved the video *The Lion King*. Her favorite part was when the three friends, Simba, Pumbaa, and Timon, played in the jungle together. She had learned how to use the remote and would rewind the tape again and again so she could watch that part over and over. She would dance as the video ran and could imitate the animated figures exactly with her movements. We actually asked the parents to bring the video in after lunch, so as to watch her do this. She was amazingly accurate.

She was very particular about what foods she would eat. She had been very late to get off baby foods and still, if a food was rough like a cracker or crunchy like celery or nuts, she refused it. She preferred "easy" foods like bananas, tapioca, and macaroni and cheese.

Holly went to sleep without complaint at bedtime but she needed to rock back and forth in her bed and make a noise like "NNN" in order to get herself to sleep. This usually went on for about half an hour. Sometimes when she was upset or angry, she also did this to calm herself down.

After doing our standard testing, we performed a special test on Holly that is called the PEP-R (Psychoeducational Profile). This is a test that looks at a child's abilities in a different way and incorporates within the testing some chances to teach in a "hand over hand" manner, with the examiner demonstrating testing with his or her hand holding the child's. It also involves seeing how a child reacts to certain sensations, such as feeling a pebbly surface and a smooth one. Bells are rung to gauge the child's reaction to a sudden sound in the background, whether it is under- or over-reactive, and how quickly the child notices and responds to the sound.

As I was getting Holly to walk up the stairs, she became intrigued by some empty boxes in the hallway that were waiting to be recycled.

"Gateway," she read off a box, "Gateway."

Remember, this was a child who could not talk.

As we had suspected, Holly was autistic. The person coordinating her case, Edie, took our team through a specialized questionnaire that scored Holly on various behavioral characteristics that we had observed and that her parents had reported about her actions at home. She fit many of the typical characteristics of a child with autism. She had difficulties in the ways that she communicated. She had some "scattering" of skills, some that were way behind her age level, and some, such as her reading the word on the box and remembering exactly what order her stuffed animals went in, that were way above those of an average four-year-old. She had some ritualistic behavior and became confused or agitated by changes in her routine. Though she did not demonstrate many unusual movements, the rocking at night was an example of a repetitive, calming behavior, and she had some differences in her reactions to sensations, including food.

Autism is not a problem with emotional attachment. The belief that autistic children show no affection is incorrect. They are usually very attached to their parents and to other familiar people. Nevertheless, they have difficulty sharing an experience, especially one that is confusing to them. We always look for what we call "joint attention" in a child with some of these characteristics. For example, if a "normal" child sees a clown at the circus fall over his big feet she may laugh and turn to her mother with a smile, as if saying, "Isn't this fun?" If a baby is being fed, he might take a piece of banana and offer it to his father, who slips it in his mouth. Then the baby wants the father to do it back. Then he insists on feeding the father another piece and giggles. They are taking turns in a game.

Children with autism show these behaviors at times, but considerably less often and with a poorer quality of interaction. In working with these children in a behavioral context, it is important to establish this very basic social skill by taking an activity that the child likes very much – like swinging in someone's arms – and turn it into an opportunity to share something fun. The therapist or parent would try to encourage the child to ask for another turn to swing, to share in saying "whee!" as they swing around, and then to add another activity to the game, such as finishing the game with a big hug. Then the parent tries to extend and extend the interaction more and more. He tries to interrupt the avoidant behaviors and essentially force the child to interact socially, including even blocking the child's way to get the child to indicate a desire to have him move.

Stanley Greenspan, an expert in the area of autism and a pioneer in some of the behavioral treatments for the problem, suggests that the core problem for an autistic child is the inability to form social meaning out of the stimuli in the environment.[15] Knowing how to recite the introduction to a computer game is an excellent auditory memory skill, but if one cannot interpret the words as an explanation of the game's rules, then they are just a bunch of sounds. Dancing to a video is a good motor and imitative skill, but if the child cannot understand that dancing is a way that people express joy together with movement, then she will continue to make it a ritual without any change in form.

I know of another child with autism (he is also developmentally delayed, as is frequently the case) who cannot speak beyond the two- to three-year-old level, but you can take him out into the parking lot and see a different child.

I can point to a car, and say, "What's that, Mike?"

"A 1995 Subaru," he'll tell me, pointing, too.

"How about that one?"

"It a PT Cruiser, 2000. Pretty."

He is always right. Since a car, to me, is just a conveyance that gets me from one place to another, I marvel at his ability to do this. Mike can get very agitated during medical exams and the way I calm him is to talk about cars and NASCAR drivers. But he will never be able to carry on a conversation about cars with another person and will never be able to understand the rules of driving, which involve turn-taking and courtesy. (Come to think of it, there are some non-autistic people on the road who don't understand these rules, either!)

There are many, many different treatments for autism and I have talked to numerous parents who swear by one treatment or another. Studies on many of them are inconclusive. The behavioral ones seem to work best, and it is my opinion (with some research to back it up) that the more intense the behavioral interaction, the more successful the treatment. Our psychologist offers sessions that help parents to work with their children at home, because it is parents, who already share a strong bond with their child, who can provide the most lasting interactive results.

About controversial treatments, I offer parents this advice. When considering a treatment that is not fully proven to work, ask the following questions.

Will the treatment harm the child in any way? How expensive will it be? How much will it interfere with the regular flow of our family's daily life? Will it interfere with a treatment that is better proven to work? Is it advertised as a cure-all for every problem? Be suspicious. Nothing is a cure-all.

If the answers to these questions are all satisfactory, then I would say, "Go for it." What harm can it do? For example, I tell parents that some research suggests (but does not prove to the standard that is generally scientifically accepted) that Vitamin B6 and Magnesium can be helpful in reducing the symptoms of autism. I am sure to tell them that I do not know whether it works or not. Still, who am I to keep them from doing something that might help?

The very encouraging news is that autism can improve enormously given early and intense intervention. I have seen children who appear very autistic who receive treatment, and by the time they go off to kindergarten, only a trained observer would know that they had once had that label. They may still show some differences in their behaviors, but they are very substantially reduced. This was not thought to be possible in the late 1980s or even early 1990s.

On the less encouraging side is the fact that the number of children diagnosed with autism increased practically beyond belief in the latter part of the twentieth century. A diagnosis that used to be present in 1 out of every 10,000 children is now thought to be present in about 1 out of every 500–1000 children.[16] That is a staggering jump. Although there are many theories, no one knows why it is so. It is not just the result of better diagnoses of the condition, though that is one reason for the change. All we know at the DEC is that we see an enormous number of children who have autism or many of its symptoms. All of them fall in the "autistic spectrum," which includes a condition called "pervasive developmental delay."

There is also a percentage of children who have what is known as high-functioning autism, or Asperger syndrome. (Actually, there may be some mild differences between these two diagnoses, but these distinctions are fairly technical and do not need to be addressed here.) These are children who are bright and are enormously capable in areas that interest them, but who show some of the core problems that are present in autism, including a lack of understanding of social connections.

It was many years ago when I saw the first child I was aware of with this condition and, at that time, I knew far less about autism in its subtler forms. I saw Cameron first as a small child because he had low muscle tone, a large head, and was a little behind in his gross motor skills. He was a large, soft child who was a little late to talk. Once he started talking he spoke in his own language. He called a slide "eep," and "bopm, bopm" was a ball. He also didn't seem to know how to monitor the volume of his voice, sometimes speaking much too loudly, and sometimes so quietly that no one could hear him.

After several years, though, he had stopped this and had begun using very sophisticated language. Actually, he was in some ways a little professor, since he enjoyed giving lectures on things he was interested in. He loved animals and wanted to hear any book that told anything about them, especially facts about zoo animals.

His long-suffering mother allowed him to have cages full of snakes and lizards, and Cameron spent a lot of time finding and fixing food for his pets. The family also had five cats and a dog and Cameron would cuddle and play with them for hours, which was much more time than he spent playing with his sister. He didn't get along very well with the other children in the neighborhood; he never quite seemed to understand the games they played and seemed to prefer doing things by himself. The other children also got tired of his lecturing and his quasi grown-up ways.

At age five he developed some funny movements. He would pace the floor and make explosive, sudden sounds or click his tongue and flap his fingers against his thumb. He did this several times a day, especially when he seemed stressed. When his mother asked him what he was doing, sometimes he didn't even seem aware that he was behaving strangely.

He'd look down at his hands in surprise as if they didn't even belong to him and say, "I don't know. It just makes me feel better to do this."

When I saw Cameron do this I assumed that he had Tourette syndrome, since he was showing a pattern of vocal and motor tics. After some routine tests to rule out other neurological conditions, I began him on the appropriate medication for Tourette syndrome. The behaviors improved briefly but returned in full force shortly after. After some adjustment in the medicine without improvement, I sent him to a neurologist, who also thought he had Tourette syndrome, though he said it was not quite typical. He also had no success in treating the movements.

Other things became evident when Cameron entered school. He shone in science activities but had a very difficult time with arithmetic. He just couldn't seem to understand the concepts behind addition and subtraction. He was also regularly accused of having terrible handwriting, though he really tried to make his letters properly. And he still had a lot of trouble relating to the other children. He seemed to become angry and agitated very easily when things were confusing to him.

One day, Cameron was riding his bike after school and accidentally crashed into a little girl who darted off the sidewalk and right in his path. She fell and badly hurt her arm, which turned out to be broken. As the mothers and neighbors gathered, he stood to the side, saying nothing but shaking his head over and over as if fussing at himself.

When everything had been taken care of and the girl was brought to the doctor, Cameron and his mother went home.

She gently said, "Cameron, I know you felt bad about hurting Ashley, but you didn't say you were sorry. It's very important to tell people that you're sorry when you hurt them."

Cameron told her, in obvious distress, "I know, Mom, I know. But I didn't know what tone of voice to use. If she had been an animal, I know I could have said [and here he took on the high-pitched sing-song voice we often use toward animals], 'Poor baby, I'm so-oo sorry.' But I knew that wasn't right, and I didn't know how to say it."

When I heard these stories the next time Cameron came in, it made me very suspicious that something else was going on with him. We already knew that he had learning disabilities and anger control problems, but it seemed as if all the hints and clues were pointing to something larger.

We sent Cameron to the Center of Development and Learning in Chapel Hill. After a battery of tests that took all day, a very exhausted Cameron and his mother conferred with a doctor.

"Cameron is autistic," they told her, after they had gone over his scores.

She was stunned. "Are you saying that this is a possibility or that you're sure?"

"We're sure," was the answer.

They supplied her with a lot of information about Asperger syndrome and after she had read it, she was convinced. The material also made a believer out of me.

Since that time, I have had a lot of training in recognizing and treating autism, and I now realize that Cameron's symptoms were subtle, but classic in character. I have seen many children with similar symptoms and they are not hard to pick out.

Cameron is now in high school. Partly because his mother has continued to be in his corner all through school, he has been allowed various modifications in his schoolwork. He has had a good bit of help, including a special class for a while, occupational therapy, and even a taxi to take him to a school outside of his district that better met his educational needs. He has recently started using the services of Vocational Rehabilitation, an agency that helps young adults with disabilities of various sorts to get job training and the appropriate education. He has always been bright and observant and has a very dry sense of humor.

Sometimes, however, he is funny when he doesn't mean to be. He received a birthday invitation, which included an RSVP. His mother explained that he needed to call the number and tell them that he was coming to the party. She did not realize she needed to explain further than that.

Cameron picked up the phone and dialed. When someone on the other end said, "Hello?" he said, simply, "I'm coming," and hung up the phone. His mother was sure that the person would assume she'd received an obscene phone call! She had to sit him down and explain the full procedure for accepting an invitation by phone.

"Sometimes he understands situations right away, but then, other times when you think he would understand, he doesn't," she says. "He takes everything so literally. I'm sure if I said 'let's hit the road,' Cameron would be looking for a stick. But he does have a great sense of humor when *he* makes the joke!"

Cameron had to take the test for his driver's permit four times before he passed. He was thrilled that he could finally drive, or so he thought. In fact, during the actual driving lessons at school, he terrified the driving instructor so much that he made him stop the car several times and he never allowed him on the highway as he did the other teenagers. The instructor told his mother that he had passed Cameron because he was older than the other kids and had tried so hard, but that he was a driving hazard and should have much more practice before he was actually put behind the wheel. He is clumsy, begins his unusual hand movements when he gets anxious in the car, and he has trouble with the communication and directions from the adult in the front seat with him. His mother is not planning for him to get his license for quite some time.

Cameron is hoping to have his own zoo when he is grown. In fact, many people with high-functioning autism do very well professionally as adults if they work on a specific interest of theirs. Temple Grandin, who has written several books on being autistic, is an example. She also loves animals and has designed and manufactured new equipment that is more humane for animals and is now used widely.[17]

From what I have read, I suspect that Thomas Edison may have had a mild form of high-functioning autism. When he was born, people thought he might be abnormal because his head was so large in proportion to his body. He got into all sorts of trouble as a small child because of "experiments" that showed minimal understanding of the consequences of his actions. For example, at age six, he set a fire inside his father's barn "just to see what it would do." What happened, of course, was that the barn burned down to the ground. Fortunately, no one was injured.

At about the same time, he went with a friend to swim in a small creek on the outskirts of town. The way Edison described the event as an adult was as follows.

After playing in the water a while, the boy with me disappeared in the creek. I waited around for him to come up but as it was getting dark I concluded to wait no longer and went home. Some time in the night I was awakened and asked about the boy. It seems the whole town was out with lanterns and had heard that I was last seen with him.[18]

No one in the town could figure out why Edison didn't tell anyone that the boy had drowned, or if he even understood that the boy had drowned. It may have been that, like Cameron, he didn't know exactly how to tell what had happened, what emotions were appropriate, and may not have entirely understood the significance behind the event. Some people in town called him a boy "without feelings." It may have been more that he was a boy for whom feelings were a confusing world that he didn't quite have the key to interpreting, even though he had them.

Edison had a great deal of difficulty in school learning the work in the way that it was taught there. The teachers thought him feebleminded. Eventually his mother took him out of school and taught him at home, basically by giving him books to read and letting him follow his own direction, guided by what he found fascinating. He never learned to spell or write very well.

Clearly, Edison found his own niche as he grew older, but he still had some very unusual behaviors and characteristics. While obsessed with a scientific problem, he was known to spend up to 60 hours without food, sleep, or much to drink in order to continue experimenting. He forced the people who worked for him to do the same. Perhaps he did not understand that not everyone felt the way he did about his work.

On one occasion, he had been notified that if he did not pay his real-estate taxes immediately, he would be fined an additional fee. He went to city hall to pay and, while standing in a long line, began thinking about a scientific problem related to multiplex telegraphy. Suddenly he found himself at the front of the line, with the officer collecting the taxes asking him his name so he could find Edison's bill. Edison stared at him blankly.

"I don't know it, sir," he was forced to reply.[19]

The man furiously ordered him to step out of line. Edison could not pay the bill until he remembered his name and ended up having to pay the extra fee.

Odd behavior, to say the least. Yet he was one of the most prolific achievers of the twentieth century, if not of all time. We use his inventions numerous times daily and could hardly do without them, as anyone who has been in a power failure can attest to.

I once went to a conference on autism where a young man with high-functioning autism spoke about his life. He was an exceptionally good speaker, funny, interesting, and very enthusiastic. Anyone listening to him might have thought, "What is wrong with him? He seems fine!", until the question-and-answer period came. When the ideas and thoughts were coming from other people and not spouting from himself, he seemed at a loss. This intelligent young man suddenly stammered and answered inappropriately and often said that he didn't understand the question. One can imagine what a serious problem this inability to carry on an appropriate conversation could be, and it was easy to understand why he had a great deal of trouble keeping a job or developing friendships. It was touching but sad when he handed around his favorite teddy bear to show the audience how cute it was.

I hope that in the near future we will be able to discover the core problem, either neuroanatomic, chemical, or toxic, that is the key to autism so we can find better ways to prevent and cure it. However, this begs the question: Would we have Thomas Edisons if we did find a cure? And what would the person with high-functioning autism prefer? And if we cured someone like Edison, would we do away with that highly focused drive in their area of expertise? Or would they be able to incorporate both that drive and the ability to form better social relationships?

Oliver Sacks says in the preface to *An Anthropologist on Mars*:

> Defects, disorders, diseases…can play a paradoxical role, by bringing out latent powers, developments, evolutions, forms of life, that might never be seen, or even be imaginable, in their absence. It is the paradox of disease, in this sense, its "creative" potential… Thus while one may be horrified by the ravages of developmental disorder or disease, one may sometimes see them as creative, too – for if they destroy particular paths, particular ways of doing things, they may force the nervous system into making other paths and ways, force on it an unexpected growth and evolution.[20]

It's food for thought.

Chapter 15

The Falling Sickness

Canst thou not minister to a mind diseased,
Pluck from the memory a rooted sorrow,
Raze out the written troubles of the brain?

William Shakespeare, Macbeth

I have a disability myself: I have seizures. Thanks to the miracles of modern medicine, I am fully functional and they currently do not bother me at all. But that wasn't always the case.

They started when I was seven years old. My family had moved that year from a smallish home in a San Juan suburb to the heart of Old San Juan to restore a beautiful old house. It was a huge project. Workmen came and went daily. The noise from the carpentry and masonry work was terribly distracting. We moved from room to room, using a hotplate to cook until the kitchen was done and often eating dinner out at a local restaurant.

After the house was done, I saw what my parents had seen in their mind's eye when they initially bought the house. It was gorgeous, and it's still the house I think of as my main childhood home. At the beginning, however, there was peeling plaster and paint to scrape off and repair, old, rotten doors and balconies to replace, and, everywhere and always, dust and chips of paint on the floor.

One morning, I woke up with a terrible stomach-ache, the worst I ever remembered having. Doubled over, I slowly made my way down the hall and up the uneven wooden stairs to my parents' room. I remember resting several times on the steps and feeling the cold wood against my stomach. I had a headache also.

"Mama?" I said.

"What is it, love?" she asked me, looking worried.

"Come lie down on the bed and tell us," said my father, patting the sheets. "Are you sick?"

"My stomach hurts really badly."

And that is the last thing I remember until I woke up briefly in the doctor's office while they were moving me onto the table to do skull X-rays. My parents told me later that I had simply seemed to fall asleep, but that I couldn't be awakened. I couldn't hear or respond to anything they said. They were terrified. My father grabbed me up in his arms and they ran out the door to the doctor, hurriedly telling my sister Kim where they were going and to call a neighbor.

I woke up again in the hospital, wearing one of those pale blue hospital gowns with no back and feeling very drowsy. My stomach still hurt, and I had a terrible headache. Everyone kept asking me how I was feeling and I felt a little confused, but kept saying, "I'm fine, I just have a headache."

I had an EEG, an electroencephalogram, to examine my brain waves. They gave me something green to drink, sweet and bitter at the same time. They put cold, paste-like glue in my hair to attach wires. Because there were some abnormal brain waves, they made a diagnosis of seizures.

The next day they brought me some pills with my disgusting breakfast of lumpy unsalted oatmeal that I pushed away. I was told I was supposed to take the pills so I would feel better, and so that I wouldn't get very, very sick. No one told me at that time that I had had a seizure. I think I was told that I was having a brain problem.

I took my pills every day, and I was allowed to go back to school in a few days. I recall that I still had a lot of bad headaches and stomach-aches and I had a lot of trouble getting up in the morning. My parents recall that I was often very irritable that year. I had always been a good student, but that next grading period, I had several low Bs and a C or two. I was quite upset and went to my teacher to ask her about it.

"Well, you know, you have been sick," she comforted me.

I found out later that the doctors had told my parents that they shouldn't expect me to do well in school anymore, so my parents had explained to my teachers to go easy on me and not expect too much, as they had been told to do. I was probably having some sedation and possibly even confusion from the medication. Fortunately, when the side effects of the medicine wore off by the next year, I went back to my regular standard of work.

Every few days, I would have some strange sensations that were very difficult to explain to my parents. I just knew they felt odd.

"It sounds like all the sounds around me are worried or something," I'd tell them. "Even the buzz of the refrigerator. Sometimes they're loud and sometimes they feel like they're coming from far away."

By the next school year, I seemed back on track, both scholastically and healthwise, though I still took my medicine faithfully three times a day.

And so it went until we moved to Canada, where we saw a new neurologist.

"When was the last time she had a seizure?" he asked.

When my mother informed him that it had been about five years, and a subsequent EEG was normal, he took me off the medication. I didn't have any further problems for a long time. I put it all behind me and didn't think of myself as having any sort of health problem at all.

Once or twice in college and several times in medical school, I had some of those same odd sensations that I had had when I was a child. I would know when they were about to happen and they made me feel weird. I consulted a doctor who said she thought they were migraine variants, since I did have the occasional migraine.

One day at medical school, I happened to be reading about lead poisoning in children. It stated the symptoms of mild, moderate, and severe lead poisoning. It stated that young children in particular were very susceptible to lead in their surroundings. As I was aware, one of the main vehicles for lead was old paint chips.

There was then a statement that read, "Lead poisoning is becoming more common in middle and upper middle class families as the interest in restoring old houses grows. The air is filled with lead dust and the children are unknowingly exposed to excessive doses of lead."

I was stunned. I realized I had experienced many of the symptoms of acute lead poisoning: headaches, stomach-aches, irritability, and seizures. In fact, I remember being fussed at for peeling the paint off the doors with my fingers. And I bit my nails. It was inevitable that I would have gotten some lead paint in my mouth. Presumably I lost a few IQ points, too, since everyone who has severe enough lead poisoning to cause a seizure, does.[21] Fortunately, it hasn't affected my life in the long run.

I wish that was the end of the story. But it isn't. About five years ago I began having weird sensations again, this time much stronger and much more frequent, even as often as ten or twelve times a day. The first time it happened, I thought I was beginning the flu.

But, to tell the truth, it wasn't really like the flu. First a wave of something rushed over me, not a hot flash, more the feeling that one gets when one is trying not to sneeze, except that it was felt all over my body and it was very unpleasant. Then I got tingling and buzzing that started at my center and spread out to my fingers, toes, and lips. Then I started getting very dizzy, sometimes so dizzy that I had to lie down.

I could be talking to a patient and have one of these spells start. I would know it was happening, but I could keep on talking in a perfectly coherent way most of the time; it was all going on inside me. I did not lose consciousness.

I went to Asheville to see a neurologist who heard my history and had an EEG and an MRI done.

He brought me the EEG.

"It's very clear, as you can see here," he said, pointing, "that you are having partial simple seizures. (These are seizures that cause strange sensations but involve no loss of consciousness). We'll need to start some medication. Not only could you lose consciousness if you allow them to continue, but they will probably get more and more frequent. That is usually the way these things go."

Oh, I thought, amazingly calm. It's what I thought it was; I'm having seizures. I drove home calmly, prescription in hand.

In the middle of the night, I woke up.

"OH MY GOD," I suddenly thought. "I'm having seizures! I have a disability that is going to be around for the rest of my life! This is not in my plans!"

It was surprisingly difficult for me to accept, especially considering that I worked with children with medical problems all the time. I guess all of us like to keep that "it won't happen to me" feeling that slightly distances us from other people with problems.

Again, I had to go through the adjustment of trying different medications, being very frequently sleepy and slightly dazed while my body got used to the anticonvulsant medication. There was a very difficult three months or so where I felt as if I walked around at home and work as a living zombie. Then one time, when I was switching from one medicine to another (and had to take both at the same time for a while), I couldn't keep my balance easily and I couldn't tell if my feet were going in the right place when I walked. Side effects of medication are one of the most irritating things about having no choice but to treat oneself.

I was eventually switched to Lamictal, one of the newer anticonvulsants. It was originally meant to be a secondary medication, for people whose seizures could not be controlled by only one medicine, but it can work very well as a single drug for some people, as well. I am fortunately one of them. I do extremely well on the medication and my odd sensations occur only very rarely. I never lose consciousness. I am religious about taking my Lamictal.

I am well aware that if I had lived even 50 years ago, I would be a chronic invalid. At Thanksgiving, when we go around the table saying what we are grateful for, I always think of Lamictal and the researchers who work to find cures for disease. I can live a completely normal life and for that, I am always indebted.

Some of my patients are not so lucky. I see several children whose disease cannot be controlled by medication and who therefore have a number of seizures a week. These children usually do very poorly. They are dazed and sleepy after their seizures, they don't learn well, and they need constant supervision and often have to wear protective head gear. I see others who are so continually sedated by their medication that they have difficulty making any further developmental progress. I even have one patient who had to have the two halves of her brain separated in order to stop the focus of the seizure from spreading. She has done astoundingly well in her development despite this.

I don't usually treat the patients' seizures myself. Their primary physician or neurologist usually takes care of the medicine. But I do often tell the parents that I also have a seizure disorder so that they know that it does not always spell doom and gloom for their child.

We see an increasing number of Hispanic patients as more legal and illegal Mexicans and Guatemalans come to the area, searching for work.

Mexico City is known for its terrible pollution, since it is so crowded and the government puts far fewer restrictions than the US government does on industrial emissions. These children, in particular, suffer all too commonly from lead poisoning. Some of them have seizures and some have other symptoms. They may also have significant learning problems. The local pediatricians are very good about checking lead levels in these children. Recent studies suggest that even a level of blood lead that we used to consider acceptable and not necessarily worth medical treatment can cause some developmental problems.[21] It's scary.

There is another situation I have seen several times where seizures have, in a different sense, caused developmental problems.

Mohammed, a kindergarten child, was sent to us in order to rule out fetal alcohol syndrome. This was extremely shameful and humiliating to his mother because of her Muslim background. Drinking is forbidden and excessive drinking, in particular, would be considered dreadful.

"I have never had any alcohol in my whole life," she told me, tearfully. "It is against my religion. But the teacher and the guidance counselor at the school don't seem to believe me."

"My son is a good boy," she continued. "He does have problems in school; I know that. But he is a dutiful son and very loving. He takes good care of his little brother and sister. He helps me in the house."

Mohammed was an interesting-looking little boy. He wore glasses on his tiny face that kept slipping off his nose because it was so small. He had wide-spaced eyes with slightly drooping eyelids. His hairline was low and his fingers were short with tiny fingernails. His upper lip was not flat and smooth like those of children with fetal alcohol syndrome, but very bowed, which gave him a cherubic look.

Although he had some features that were similar to those of children with fetal alcohol syndrome, he certainly did not have a classic presentation. His intelligence was in the borderline range, meaning that he was not developmentally delayed, but that he was a good bit behind.

It was during the interview with his mother that the clue came. Although she had cited no particular complications during her pregnancy, when I asked if anyone in the family had seizures, she said that she had had them all her life.

"Were you on medication during the pregnancy?" I asked.

"I was on Dilantin," she told me.

"Did your doctor tell you that Dilantin could be dangerous to your baby?" I asked her.

"No. He just told me that it was important for me not to have a seizure during pregnancy."

Very unfortunately, a certain percentage (studies vary, but usually suggest about 10 to 20 percent)[22] of babies exposed to anticonvulsants in fetal life develop significant problems, including unusual facial features, possible malformations of the heart, spinal cord, and kidneys, as well as learning problems. Phenytoin (Dilantin) and Valproic acid (Depakene) are the two major culprits. Of even more concern to the fetus is when the mother with seizures is on more than one anticonvulsant medication, which increases the likelihood of problems. Most obstetricians work carefully with a neurologist for their pregnant patients with seizures in order to find a safer medication that is effective and to decrease the number of anticonvulsants being taken. Folic acid taken before and during pregnancy is also preventative[23]. The most important thing is keeping the mother from having a seizure, which can also be dangerous to the baby.

Of course, the safest course is to change a woman to another medication when she is trying to get pregnant, since many teratogens (drugs and viruses that affect fetuses) do their worst in the first month or two of gestation, often before a woman knows she is having a child. The reality is that it seldom happens that way. It is my opinion that all neurologists should warn their seizure patients about the risks to their babies while they are of childbearing age.

I was very fortunate that my children were half-grown by the time my seizures recurred so I never had to worry about appropriate medication during pregnancy. This is certainly a difficult decision for any woman who has a seizure disorder and wants children. None of the anticonvulsants are completely safe in pregnancy and there is no known safe dose, so each prospective mother obviously has to weigh the risk herself.

Chapter 16

Smart Mothers, Horrible Choices

On horror's head horrors accumulate;
Do deeds to make heaven weep, all earth amazed.

William Shakespeare, Othello

I met Victoria Van Dyke when she was referred to us at the University of Minnesota, during my residency. She was a child who had what is called "cyclic vomiting." She had seen a number of doctors, both her own regular physician and several private specialists. She came with her mother, each of them carrying two suitcases, as if well aware that they would be having a long stay. Her mother was very solicitous of her, fluffing her pillows, arranging her stuffed animals on the bed and the shelves, and patting her hair.

Victoria, on the other hand, seemed resigned to her stay, but not very happy. She pulled out a Ramona book and buried her head in it while her mother told us her daughter's unhappy history.

"Nobody seems to know what is causing her vomiting," she told us. "She's baffled some of the best specialists in the county. They've done all sorts of tests. Sometimes she goes for a while without any vomiting and then she'll have a week or two where she vomits after every meal. None of us know what to do about it."

She was exceptionally calm and unworried as she told us this. In fact, she seemed to take a little pride in the rarity of Victoria's disease. I have known many adults who seem to be somewhat proud of their own illnesses; we are all aware of the people who enjoy talking endlessly about their myriad illnesses to whoever will listen. We all also know people who seem to have a new ache or pain every day. But a mother who was proud of her child's sickness was more unusual.

Vicky, as she asked to be called, was an only child. Her father was a long-distance trucker and wasn't home very much, though she talked about him with obvious affection.

"When Dad comes home," she told one of the medical students, "we do lots of fun stuff. So long as I'm not sick. We went to the State Fair last month. It was awesome – all those animals and exhibits and stuff. I ate about a zillion Tom Thumb doughnuts and that time I didn't throw up! My Mom fussed at him for letting me eat whatever junk I wanted, but I liked it."

However, Vicky's father was on a trip to California and we didn't see him during her hospitalization.

The first night, about half an hour after her meal, Vicky turned pale and ran quickly to the bathroom and vomited.

"She's doing it again," said her mother, rolling her eyes. "This is what our life is like. I hardly ever have any time to myself."

She and the medical student assigned to Vicky, Jennifer, became very friendly. Mrs. Van Dyke was very willing to talk and showed interest in Jennifer's life, too. She asked Jennifer a lot of questions about how she had decided to become a doctor. In fact, they seemed to be getting along so well that she invited Jennifer to come out to dinner with her.

Jennifer came back the next morning, bubbling over with enthusiasm about her dinner the night before.

"She is so nice," she exclaimed. "We went to this really nice restaurant that served really good Italian food. And she treated, which was great, since I probably couldn't even afford breadsticks at that fancy a place. We talked about all sorts of things."

"It's nice that she can get away sometimes," she said. "She's such a good mom. She practically never leaves Vicky's side."

And it was true. Mrs. Van Dyke did come out to talk to the nurses, but usually she was there taking care of Vicky, holding her head when she vomited, cleaning her up. She was really a little too overprotective.

She also had lengthy conversations with the doctors about Vicky's condition. She was very knowledgeable about various medical tests. She had read a great deal about the causes of cyclic vomiting.

"Do you think that the upper GI [gastrointestinal] should be repeated? The radiologist said it was inconclusive."

One of the tests we did on Vicky was a screen for toxins and medications. Other hospitals had also done this, but the tests had come back negative. This test came back positive for ipecac. Ipecac is a medicine that is used to induce vomiting. In large doses, or dosing over a long period of time, it can be very dangerous.

That certainly focused the direction of our diagnosis of what was causing Vicky's vomiting.

From near the beginning of the time that we had met Vicky and her mother, we had suspected or, at least, considered the possibility of a mental illness called Munchausen by proxy. This has become somewhat more familiar to the general public recently because there has been more media attention paid to it and also because of the movie *The Sixth Sense*, which portrayed a mother who was secretly poisoning her child.

Munchausen by proxy is a situation in which, for secondary gain, a parent secretly causes his or her child to become ill. The vast majority of the parents who do this are mothers. The classic pattern is that they have a distant husband who is not fulfilling their need for attention, a history of mental health problems in the past, and they are trying to gain attention and recognition in the role of self-sacrificing, devoted mother of a chronically ill child. They seem to enjoy pulling the wool over people's eyes, and not infrequently also engage in petty thievery.

Frequently the diseases described are things that happen intermittently, such as vomiting, apnea (breathing stoppages), and seizures. In that way, a report that it happened at home is hard to argue with. Sometimes, the doctor will hospitalize the child and prevent the mother from being with the child without supervision to see if the episodes still occur.

Obviously, this behavior is incredibly difficult to prove. Even when we found the ipecac in Vicky's system, we had no evidence that it had been given to her by her mother. Eventually, with Vicky's testimony, we were able to prove this and Vicky went to live with relatives.

There are some classic behaviors to watch for that, once you have seen them, stand out like a sore thumb. These mothers have a different air about them when they are describing their children's diseases. They seem surprisingly matter-of-fact, almost as if they were discussing an interesting case at medical rounds. They also seem to enjoy describing their own dramatic (and sometimes fictitious) illness. Once a mother proudly told me that she had to sleep with an apnea monitor because sometimes she stopped breathing while asleep.

"Really?" I asked, incredulously.

"Really, truly," she laughed. "It's keeping me alive."

I told a colleague about this and he asked, "If she has stopped breathing and the monitor goes off, who is going to start her breathing again?"

I remembered that she and her husband had separated about a year before.

"Uh, good question," I agreed. "I have no idea."

Another interesting behavior that is common in these mothers is that they develop a very close relationship with medical professionals in order to make them their allies. Mrs. Van Dyke, Vicky's mother, not only took to dinner the medical student who would be taking care of her daughter but also helped out the nurses and got to know them individually.

I know of another mother whom a doctor colleague of mine accused of deliberately putting infectious material in her child's ears in order to continue to cause ear infections. She had a good bit of proof that this had occurred, and testified against the mother in court. Nevertheless, the mother still sent her a singing Valentine on Valentine's Day and continued to take her daughter to that doctor for her pediatric care. My colleague couldn't understand it.

The classic Munchausen by proxy mother is astonishingly knowledge-able about all the details and nuances of the disease her child seems to have. One mother gave me a whole file folder with articles about her daughter's problem, laughing and saying that she had done a research paper on it for her night class. A surprising number of the mothers have had some sort of medical training: they are nurses, radiology technicians, were premed in college and then dropped out, and so forth. Of course, this is not always the case. Many have just read up on a lot of illnesses. Usually the child has been to a number of doctors and the family is still "doctor-shopping."

They come across as exceptionally dedicated mothers, very protective of their children. I know one who used to argue incessantly with the child's teacher that he wasn't getting his medicine at exactly the minute he was supposed to get it. The medicine was touted by the mother to be for diabetes. In fact, I found out by legally obtaining the medical records from the endocrinologist that the child had been worked up for "diabetes insipidus," which is different from the insulin-deficient diabetes most people are familiar with and which the school thought she had. The medicine she was on was for diabetes insipidus. Furthermore, the work-up for the diabetes insipidus was negative, though that was not generally known. People have no reason not to believe a parent who says that her child has a certain disease and needs a certain medicine, especially if they say that the doctor said the child had the disease.

The same mother packed her son a special lunch every day because she said he was allergic to so many different foods. One mother (described in a medical journal) who was faking her children's near-fatal episodes of Sudden Infant Death Syndrome (SIDS) was even the respected leader of a support group for SIDS parents.

But that's what makes this mental illness so complicated to ferret out: sometimes children really *do* have multiple food allergies, diabetes, SIDS and other major problems! So Munchausen by proxy can be diagnosed only through very careful observation of the family's patterns of behavior, and the diagnosis cannot be made with absolute certainty without some sort of proof that the parent is causing the problem. With police permission, mothers' pocketbooks have been searched surreptitiously for drugs that cause diarrhea or vomiting, and hidden video cameras have been used to try to collect evidence from hospital rooms. Sometimes these attempts are successful and there have been several reports of hidden cameras showing mothers smothering their babies with pillows in order to cause an apnea spell.

I become suspicious if there are several children in a family who all have some sort of different rare disease. If one has apnea (stops breathing), another has three types of complex seizures, a third has chronic, unexplained diarrhea, and the mother herself has hypoglycemia, I start to be skeptical. It's one thing if everyone in the family has the same rare disease, but quite another for everyone to be sick in a different way. In one case like this, I was able to prove that the diseases were not real. In several others, I had no proof at all and was unable to do anything, although I would report it to Protective Services. Doctors and other professionals are required to report even suspicion without proof of any type of abuse. When Protective

Services receive a report of this sort, they frequently investigate it only cursorily because of their limited knowledge of the condition and the very vague nature of the abuse. It's understandable when they have so many other serious and obvious cases.

This problem can be like the proverbial "elephant in the living room" used to describe families with an alcoholic, that no one admits to. It is unusual for the father to know what is happening but often several siblings are involved and they don't, or can't, seem to tell. There was a fascinating and horrifying article in *Pediatrics* that was written by an adult survivor of a mother with Munchausen by proxy.[24] The mother would actually smash her daughter's bones with a hammer in order to break them and then inject her with material to infect the bones. And all the while, the mother never talked to the child about what she was doing. The doctors were baffled as to why the child kept breaking bones and why the fractures did not heal, and the girl was somehow convinced she must keep silent about what was happening.

Finally, when the mother began doing the same thing to another sibling, her daughter told her that she would tell if her mother ever did it again, and this stopped the mother's abuse. Though apparently not able to protect herself, the child could not bear the thought of her brother undergoing the same torture.

It's a very strange world out there. People do things that are so bad and so crazy that it is hard to believe that such behavior is possible. However, Munchausen by proxy is more common than one might think, though not usually as blatant and severe as the case just described.

What constitutes child abuse? Obviously poisoning a child or smothering a baby with a pillow are cases of severe abuse. But is it abuse to pretend that one's child has an illness when the child doesn't? Is it abuse to give a medicine to a child who doesn't need it? How about a mother who checks her child for diabetes every time the father draws his own blood because the mother is worried the child may also have the illness? I have seen all these things. How does this compare in severity to the situation of a child who is being verbally abused with curses and constant putdowns? (In such cases it is also very hard to remove a child from home, although verbal abuse can do irreparable harm.) How do these behaviors compare to a Jehovah's Witness who refuses to have a transfusion for a child who has severely lost blood?

How about a person who refuses to have his or her child immunized (sometimes with intelligent arguments to support the decision)? Some of these actions I would consider abuse and some I wouldn't, while others I would classify as borderline cases.

Each case must be considered on its own and the benefits of removal of the child weighed against the trauma of separation from familiar loved ones and the security of home. There is no doubt that, if possible, the best option is to stop the behaviors, if they are considered harmful to the child, through education and parent supervision.

We have to get a driver's license, a hunting license, and a pilot's license, but there is no license required for raising children. There isn't even a required course in school on how to care for and discipline children appropriately. Maybe this is something that would make a difference in the treatment of the next generation's children.

And the training can't possibly start too early. When Alex, my son, was in sixth grade, another sixth-grader showed his classmates pictures of a very cute baby.

The teacher also looked at the photos.

"Oh, how sweet," she said. "Is that your baby sister?"

"No," he said. "It's my daughter." The mother of the child, it turned out, was 17. The father was 12 and well into puberty.

Is that child abuse? And if so, which child is being abused?

Incidentally, there are some shocking statistics that indicate that previous sexual abuse is a large predictor of teenage pregnancy. In 1994, the Alan Guttmacher Institute did a study that found that 74 percent of girls who had sex before age 14 and 60 percent of those who had sex before 15 reported a history of previous sexual abuse. Also, among girls who have given birth by age 15, 39 percent of the fathers are aged 20–29.[25] That's undocumented statutory rape.

The most alarming statistic of all, from a 1992 study published by Boyer and Fine in *Family Planning Perspectives*, is that among pregnant and parenting teens, 66 percent reported previous sexual abuse and 44 percent reported previous rape. The average age for the first rape was 13.3 and the rapist's average age was 22.6.[26]

In other words, we don't necessarily have a crisis of wild and irresponsible teens. We have a crisis of victimized teens who have been sexualized early and have been exposed to violence against their bodies.

Those of us who are on the front lines fighting against the medical, physical, and sexual abuse of children need to continue to be vigilant, active, and vocal in their protection.

Chapter 17

The Deaf: A Different Culture

I have often regretted my speech, never my silence.

Anon.

Not too long ago, I traveled from North Carolina to British Columbia for my high-school reunion. I had a bit of a cold and my ears had that slightly stuffed-up feeling that one can get with a cold.

I had to change flights three times in order to get to Vancouver. Each time the plane took off and landed, I thought my ears were going to explode. When I reached my destination, I realized that I couldn't hear much at all out of one ear and less than usual out of the other.

I had a great time seeing my old high-school buddies and reminiscing after 20 years, but the one horrible experience was the cocktail party, which was held in a large, echoing room where a hundred people were talking. I realized that everything was just one big muffled buzz to me; even when people spoke directly to me, I couldn't distinguish any words. When I wanted to talk to someone, I had to beckon them outside.

This experience gave me a hint about what it would be like to be hearing impaired. Fortunately, an otolaryngologist (ear, nose, and throat doctor) back in North Carolina was able to treat me with a course of antibiotics and steroids to get rid of the infection and residual fluid I had accumulated behind my eardrum.

I noticed that the ear doctor had letters from children all over his walls that said something along the lines of, "Thank you, thank you, Dr. DeFreitas! You fixed my ears! You are a good doctor!" Most of them were accompanied by a picture of the child, smiling from ear to ear. I knew just how they felt. I wrote him a similar letter myself, as a joke, also with a picture, but I warned him that he had better not put it up on his wall!

As it happens, our DEC is located on the beautiful campus of the Morganton North Carolina School for the Deaf (NCSD). There is room for us there because, as more deaf children are assimilated into regular classrooms, the NCSD is needed less and less. Better hearing aids and cochlear implants are to a large part responsible for this change, as are attitudes towards the deaf community.

We are housed in the first floor of a building that used to be a dormitory. We have made it very cheerful: the white walls are stenciled with dinosaurs and cars and hung with pictures of storybook characters and animals. Still, it remains what it is: a long, long hall with dorm rooms – now offices – on either side of it. My office is at the end of this hall, which means I get a lot of exercise walking to the records room and waiting room, which are half a football field away.

The children love to run and kick a ball down this hall. They also love the fact that my office contains a bathtub (never used) beside the sink. I know they enjoy imagining that when all the children have left I sneak in and take a bath before I go home.

Another interesting thing about being at NCSD is that students are housed on the second and third floors of our building. Since they are deaf, they have absolutely no idea how much noise they make, yelling and moving furniture. Sometimes we hear all sorts of strange noises coming from above us and have no idea what's going on. Lucy, the social worker, seems to have people arranging furniture over her head every day.

It's fun to see a group of teenagers walking on campus signing furiously to each other and then breaking up into laughter. Whether you can understand sign language or not, you know they're cutting up and telling dirty jokes just like any other group of teenagers.

American Sign Language is interesting because some of the signs so clearly indicate their root of origin from an earlier era. "Boy" is shown by touching the rim of a cap (I guess it should now be done with the rim in the back!) and "girl" is the bonnet string against the cheek. To "lead" or "direct" is an imitation of holding a horse's reins.

We all have learned some sign language in order to communicate with our NCSD neighbors and with the various people who come into the DEC asking for directions. I am in particular very good at "I'm sorry. I can't sign," and also "Please sign more slowly." Each of us has a personal sign for his or her name. Mine is "Mama doctor."

Our speech pathologist, Nadine, and one of our psychologists have both worked at NCSD in the past and sign fluently, and they help us to interpret when we see a child or family member who is deaf. However, not everyone is fluent when they just start working at the deaf school. A parent of one of our patients used to work with deaf adolescents who had behavior problems. She essentially learned to sign as she went. And sometimes she made screamingly funny mistakes. Taking the curved fingers of the hand and running it down in front of your chest means "hungry." Whenever it was near lunchtime, she would run her hands down her chest several times, and indicate, "I'm hungry!" Unfortunately, when you use this sign in this manner more than once, it doesn't mean hungry, it means sexually aroused. She kept wondering why they laughed at her being hungry.

Once a woman came to our office to ask how to get somewhere on campus. She signed and asked if any of us were deaf. When we said no, she indicated her sympathy.

"There are so many good jokes in sign language if you're deaf," she signed. "You don't know what you're missing!"

Then she proceeded to tell one that none of us, even the people who signed well, understood. She must be right about the jokes; we certainly couldn't tell what we were missing, but I think I'll keep the privilege of hearing music in exchange.

Deaf people have a culture all unto themselves. Because they can't get each other's attention by sound, they often hit in order to get someone to pay attention to them. Some tend to be abrupt and discourteous by hearing culture standards. In fact, they don't mean to be rude at all, just brief and direct. Many deaf activists also strongly believe in "deaf pride" and the idea of a tight-knit community within, but not dependent on, the hearing world. They feel it should not be considered a handicap to be deaf and do not see any reason to learn to lip read, speak, get a cochlear implant or even a hearing aid in order to overcome the condition (assuming one or more of these steps would even be appropriate, which they sometimes aren't).

There is an equally vocal (so to speak) group who are working very hard for more inclusion of the hearing impaired in the regular school system. The North Carolina deaf schools are in danger of closing in order to reduce the budget deficit and also to encourage inclusion and a "least restrictive environment" for these students. This could work even for students who are completely deaf if an interpreter was provided. Nevertheless, many alumni feel that the deaf school provides a haven for the hearing impaired and that it serves a wide variety of needs that would not all be met in a mainstream situation.

Some recent studies do indicate that a cochlear implant, if the children fit the criteria for one, is of enormous benefit in fitting into the hearing world. The criteria include that children have not significantly improved their hearing with hearing aids and that they are of normal intelligence. If these children get their cochlear implants before they turn three, a large percentage are talking and understanding normally – yes, normally! – by kindergarten.[27] That is a pretty impressive result by anyone's standards.

As medicine continues to advance, it may very well be that almost all hearing impairments will be curable. Then these various arguments about what is best for the deaf population will likely become less pressing.

Chapter 18

Brothers and Sisters

I think they love him more than me.

Sibling of a child with developmental delay

We often like it when the brothers and sisters of patients accompany them to our office. In many cases, they can be enormously helpful in getting their siblings to show what they can do or coaxing them to cooperate. Many brothers and sisters have served as helpmate and interpreter to their special-needs siblings for years. Most are proud of doing it. To others it can be a burden. It is a surprisingly tricky job to be the "normal one."

As I have said, when I was a child, children with disabilities were not as accepted or as conspicuous as they are today. People sometimes spoke in whispers about someone who had a mentally retarded child, and these children participated far less in community activities. Those of my friends who had brothers or sisters who were disabled did not talk about it a great deal, or briefly stated that they had a "special" sibling who went to a "special" school. I know many of them felt embarrassed bringing their friends to their houses to visit because of their brother or sister.

Certainly, the majority of brothers and sisters of a child with special needs learn through poignant experience the importance of love and compassion. I think this is illustrated best by the large number of these siblings who go into caring for the special-needs population as a career. But compassion isn't always learned easily.

I had a friend in high school, Sarah, whose younger sister Helen was developmentally delayed. The family was educated and well-to-do and went way beyond what was typical then in order to try to get the best possible schooling for Helen, and gave enormously of their time and energy to help her.

The oldest boy in the family was "the smart and responsible one." He was the one who took care of Helen, defended her from other children when they were young, and was consulted in decisions to be made about her. He was also the one who was expected to do well in school and take over the family business.

My friend Sarah, the middle child, sometimes felt that there was no role left for her. Because she was closer to Helen's age, she was supposed to play with Helen and include her in her games with friends. Her older brother added to the criticism if she did not live up to perfect playmate standards that were required by her family.

Because Helen needed so much attention, Sarah often felt that there wasn't much left for her. She also seemed to live in the shadow of her high-achieving older brother. Though the brother almost seemed to go out of his way to tell people that he had a sister who was mentally retarded, Sarah was very quiet about it. She was also quiet about her quite respectable academic achievement. When she got into a very good college, there was little fanfare. Her older brother was doing very well at another prestigious college and she was simply following in his footsteps.

It was not until she left home and went to college in another province that Sarah felt that she could shake off the feeling of being the one who didn't belong and wasn't really needed in her family. She went into a profession completely unrelated to the family business and is happy and successful, with a family of her own. I do not know what her relationship with her sister is like at present, but I would bet that she still feels some resentment towards her and towards the rest of the family.

We see a lot of young people like Sarah, brothers and sisters of special-needs kids who are trying to figure out their place in their families.

One day I went on a home visit to see a child who had recently returned from a very lengthy stay in the hospital. The little boy, about 20 months, had been playing in the yard. His mother (there was no father in the picture) ran in to answer the phone and was back in less than two minutes. She searched for her son frantically and quickly found him lying face down in the neighbor's baby pool. Resuscitation brought his heartbeat back, but he had been starved of oxygen and had sustained a good bit of damage to his organs and brain. Home after three months of hospitalization, he still required round-the-clock nursing care.

I examined the little boy, Robbie, carefully and did some simple developmental testing. It was truly pitiful to see that tiny child lying there with feeding tubes, monitors, an eggshell mattress to prevent bedsores, a nurse working his stiff arms and legs, surrounded by all manner of stuffed animals and get-well cards that he hardly noticed.

But it was not he who wrung my heart the most. There was another little boy in the room, Dusty, his four-year-old brother. He was crouched in the corner watching everything and playing with a Buzz Lightyear action figure. I smiled at him several times. He smiled back and inched a little closer. I made a silly face at him. He inched still closer. Soon his hand was reaching for mine.

When I was able during the interview and exam, I made some simple conversation with him, asking if he had seen the movie *Toy Story* and commenting on his outfit.

"Would you like to see me do tricks on my tricycle?" he asked me.

"Not right now, Dusty," said his mom. "Dr. Hays is trying to look at Robbie."

His face dropped, the joy gone. He nodded and retreated back to his corner. I couldn't bear it.

"Dusty," I said. "I'll be 15 minutes more. Then I would like very much to see you ride your trike."

"Okay!" He ran outside to practice.

Afterwards, I made certain I took the time to watch him ride down a little wooden ramp he had made from a piece of plywood and to bump his trike down the two front steps of the modest house in which they lived.

"Do you like that?" he asked me after each little performance.

"I think it's just wonderful. You are so good at that!" I told him.

"Just see this one now," he'd say. "Just one more trick."

As I left I asked his mother whether he was in any sort of preschool program.

"No. I don't really have time to take him. I have to give all my energy to Robbie right now. And there's not really anyone in the neighborhood his age to play with."

She sighed and her shoulders sagged.

"I wish there was something I could do. I know he gets bored, but I just don't have the time to spend with him."

We were able to arrange some funds to pay for Dusty to get a ride to pre-school. I'm sure this has helped. Still, I worry about him and children in his situation. Not only do they have the grief involved in essentially losing a sibling, but also they can lose their parents, as well. I hope that at some point Dusty's mother was able to divide her time and to understand that she might see irreparable damage done to two children if Robbie became her only focus.

For some years I saw a boy, Fred, who was one of two children in the family. He and his older brother were only a year apart in age. He had ADHD and significant learning disabilities in reading and memory that were affecting his school performance to the point where he had been held back a year. I treated him for the ADHD and saw him regularly for medication follow-up.

Fred was effeminate, and he had unusual interests for a ten-year-old boy: he loved to cook, he spent hours building model houses, and he thought he might be an interior decorator when he grew up. I suspected, though of course, I did not know, that he was gay, and I worried about what he would have to face from the other kids when he hit high school. Hatred of homosexuality seems to me to be one of the most prevalent and virulent of society's remaining prejudices, and its victims, many of them youngsters, really suffer.

Fred's brother, Martin, was exceptionally bright. He read voraciously and was in the gifted program at school. Unfortunately, he was not gifted when it came to compassion, at least not toward his brother. He was continually putting Fred down, making fun of his hobbies, and tattling on him.

Admittedly, Fred could be annoying. He talked non-stop, seemed to have no understanding of the value of developing protective coloration (for example, he would say that his favorite color was fuchsia and not realize that most people would consider that unusual in a ten-year-old boy), and he was athletically inept. In fact, Fred's father was somewhat ashamed of him, too, and would nag him to act more masculine. He couldn't stand to see Fred concocting something delicious in the kitchen.

The fact that they were close to the same age served only to accent the difference between the boys and their capabilities.

Their mother was very aware of these family dynamics and her natural response was to jump to Fred's defense and overprotect him. Though I was sympathetic with her, this did not help the situation at all. Both Martin and their father accused her of not letting Fred grow up and always taking his side. Fred would regularly run to his mother for protection instead of defending himself. He had a tendency to get attention by acting babyish and his mother did not discourage this.

I liked Fred a lot and could see that he had all sorts of skills and aptitudes that would serve him well as an adult. How often I want to say to children who are in some way different from the pack (and how often I have said to my own kids): "I promise you that when you are an adult, some of these characteristics that your peers tease you about will be admired, and you will find a special place where you are needed. The hard part is getting through the hell of growing up before you can find that place."

In Fred's case, I wanted to say, "Look – when you're 18, move to New York or San Francisco. Attend cooking or design school, find a partner and a community of friends, and you'll be a smashing success!" Maybe one day when he's older, if he does turn out to be gay, I will say this to him.

I encouraged counseling for Fred's family, and they agreed. Although things did not improve overnight, Fred's mother did learn to stop babying him and fighting his battles for him, Martin tried to leave the room when Fred was getting on his nerves instead of verbally attacking him, and the father learned to stop picking on Fred for his quasi-feminine behavior. By no means did they always succeed, but life got a little better for everyone. Fred also found a good friend, a girl, to hang out with who considered him her boyfriend, which made the kids at school lay off him a little bit. The girl was a little domineering, but, in Fred's case, that was good because she helped him with his homework and made sure that he stayed on top of his assignments.

The trick in the years to come will be keeping Fred in school long enough to graduate. I hope it can be done. Perhaps an understanding art or home-economics teacher can help him achieve this important goal.

Isaiah, the second oldest in a family of four children, was referred to us by his third-grade teacher because of his symptoms of anxiety. He cried easily over little things, he frequently complained of headaches, he missed a lot of school, and was frequently tardy. He often asked if he could go home.

The teacher had noticed that he would tell her he felt sick when he seemed especially worried about something and that if she simply encouraged him to calm down, he would usually feel better and be able to get through the day.

We also discovered that Isaiah had initially had a hard time coming to kindergarten and cried for the first six weeks, wanting to go home.

We had seen his two brothers and his sister in the past. His siblings all had learning problems and, in fact, two of them were mildly developmentally delayed. We had not tested his parents, but it was fairly clear that they had major learning problems. Both worked at very menial jobs, and they had a lot of difficulty expressing themselves clearly and understanding what we told them.

Isaiah, although polite and pleasant, did seem anxious. His eyebrows slanted down in a worried frown, he bit his nails past the quick, and he kept wanting to check on his parents in the waiting room. We always invite parents to be in the room or watch our sessions through a one-way window, but in Isaiah's case they stayed up front to watch their younger children.

He seemed to calm down once he had a chance to see that his parents and the rest of his family was fine. Once he told us, "I need to go check to see if Dakota has had his medicine. I think Daddy brought it."

In a few minutes, he came back, looking relieved.

"Daddy brought it. I got Dakota some juice. He can't take medicine without juice."

Isaiah's IQ was in the high average range, about 113. He scored well in academic achievement and his language skills were adequate.

I asked him to draw a picture of his family. I don't want to make too much of children's drawings as the key to all their emotions, but they can be quite telling, especially if the child explains them afterwards.

Isaiah drew himself in the middle of his family, holding hands with his two brothers. His baby sister was positioned sort of hanging over his head. The figures were all very large and, as he had left his parents until last, there was no room for them.

"Do you want another piece of paper to draw your mom and dad?" I asked.

"That's okay," he said. "They're at work so I'm at home with the others."

What became evident was that Isaiah was by far the brightest member of his family. At the age of eight, he was the head of the household. He made sure his mother remembered to buy groceries, the younger children got to their doctor appointments, and that his father cashed his checks from work. The reason he was getting so anxious at school is because he was terrified that the rest of the family would fall apart without him. He was being forced to take on burdens that no child should have to bear.

It is not unusual for children with school phobia to be more worried about what is going on at home without them than actually to be scared of school.[28] Isaiah's case was not the first time that we had seen weighty responsibilities given to a small child because of family circumstances. In several cases where a mother had given her life to drugs and alcohol, we have seen four-year-olds who change their siblings' diapers, get the formula mixed, and rock the baby in the night.

One such child and her little sister were adopted, and the new mother had to gently take over the older sister's role as caretaker, without making her feel unneeded. The four-year-old child loved the care and attention she received from her adoptive mother, but it took a while for her to relinquish her need to protect (and even to discipline!) the baby. That was all she had ever known. She needed to learn how to be a child again.

Anyway, a social worker was arranged to help train Isaiah's parents to take better care of their children. I am sure Isaiah is still looking after them all, though. He will probably worry about them all his life.

An 11-year-old girl whose brother is a patient of mine wrote this essay for school:

> My brother's name is Tobias. He is two years older than me, but he looks more little. He has a handicap, he is mentally retarded and doesn't grow well. I have to take care of him a lot and so do my Mom and Dad.
>
> Sometimes I get mad at Tobias because he takes my stuff and sometimes breaks it. I used to get mad because my parents spent so much time taking him to doctors' appointments and didn't get to go to my dance recitals every time. Now I understand more that he is special and needs more attention. Even if I don't always like it.
>
> I love Tobias a lot most of the time. He and I like to bake cookies together and he laughs a lot when I play tricks. He likes it when I play the piano. We can be good friends. When he grows up, I hope we will still be friends together.

Chapter 19

Being Gifted: A Mixed Blessing

If I get a lot of awards at school, my mother and my teacher think it's great, but the other kids hate me. So sometimes I make mistakes on purpose so they won't think I'm weird.

Ten-year old patient

Children who are exceptionally intelligent or have some extraordinary talent tend to develop protective coloration so that their peers will not pick on them. Even being a good student teaches kids to be wary of their peer group. I can remember a time in seventh grade when I made a comment in class, and the girl beside me turned to me and said, "You just said that because you knew you were using a word that we didn't know and that you would look good."

In fact, I hadn't known that the other kids wouldn't know what the word I had just used meant. I remember turning red and snapping, "I did not!" which just made the other students laugh.

I also remember a drama teacher who gave me a C+ one semester, and as he handed me back my report card, which otherwise had As, he said smugly, "Ruined your report card, didn't I?" It was clear that he had never overcome his feelings of dislike for students who did better than he had in school. In fact, he clearly showed his admiration of the "cool" kids in the class.

The gifted child, like the child with learning difficulties, faces problems. But the attitude usually taken by society and, in turn, by the schools, is that these children will manage. Undoubtedly, it is assumed, they will end up on top, so it is not as important to nurture their talents as it is to help children with learning problems.

I agree that, given a limited amount of money, it is more important to work with the children who have trouble learning, but I still think that very gifted children are shortchanged. I would like to see a lot more time devoted to meeting their needs and dealing with their problems. This wouldn't have to require a lot of money. Members of the community could be used to come share their expertise with children who would most benefit, and more challenging material could be offered within the classroom. A lot of schools manage their gifted children's needs by giving them more work than everyone else and grading them more strictly, which is not really fair. Their work should be different but not increased in volume.

It is unusual for us to see a child who is exceptionally intelligent, since our focus is children who are behind in their development in some way, but it is always interesting when we do. Sometimes we are the first people to discover how intelligent a child is. I remember one eight-year-old who came to see us because of elective mutism. Elective mutism is a condition when the child is perfectly able to talk, and may talk in certain settings, but usually chooses not to do so. Nothing is better suited to hiding intelligence.

Carter was as silent as stone. His teachers at school despaired; his written work was impeccable and his end-of-grade tests indicated that he had mastered all the material, and then some. However, ever since he started kindergarten, he had not uttered one word to anyone. He shrugged and pointed and gave a rare smile but not even the other children had ever heard him speak.

At recess, he would sometimes join in on team sports but usually he sat by himself under a tree or wrote in his notebook. When the teachers told him he had to join in the play, he would, but he hung on the sides as much as he could.

Carter talked at home to his parents, though he was generally very quiet, and he talked to his brothers and sisters. In fact, his parents didn't seem to be very worried about him.

"He's not much of a talker, but when he wants to, he talks fine," said his mother, a tall and elegant African-American woman. "He's doing fine in school. I don't know why the teachers are concerned." She nervously fingered her beaded necklace.

I explained that elective mutism was often indicative of emotional problems.

"Carter," she asked him, half defensively, "is something worrying you?"

Carter shook his head and looked down.

Carter was able to do an IQ test by pointing to pictures and writing his answers down, which he didn't seem to mind too much.

The psychologist scored his test.

"I knew this was going to be high," she told us in our discussion of the child. "But guess what? – his IQ is 156! I don't think I've ever tested a kid with an IQ this high."

"Maybe he doesn't talk because he feels so alienated from the other kids in his class," suggested someone.

"Maybe. But I think there is something more to it."

His mother was very proud of his IQ score and didn't seem very surprised.

"I've always known he was really smart," she told me. "He was talking in short sentences before he was a year old."

"When did he stop talking?"

"It was somewhere after his fourth birthday, I think. Yeah, that's right. He had been sick with strep throat and when he got well again, he just stopped talking. First we thought it was because his throat was sore, but then we figured it must just be Carter. He does talk, you know. I think he's just like his father, only more so. His father has always preferred reading and watching TV to talking. I have to ask him a question several times before he answers it."

"This is not to alarm you or to suggest anything," I said. "But elective mutism can be a response to sexual abuse. Do you think there's any possibility that Carter could have been abused by anyone?"

She looked very startled.

"I can't imagine how," she said. "He is at home with us or with relatives all the time. I don't think he's ever spent the night away from home except at my sister's place. He stays over there with his cousins about once a month."

I talked to Carter, had him draw pictures for me, tried to get him to write down if anything was worrying or bothering him, but all I got was a big, fat zero. We suggested he see a psychologist regularly, but his parents decided not to do so because they felt that, since he talked at home and since many people in the family were quiet, Carter would probably just outgrow the problem. The school had him visit the guidance counselor for several months, but she, also, got nowhere.

It was not until a year later, when Carter's aunt walked in on her husband's 17-year-old son, her stepson, molesting Carter in the basement that everyone figured out what was causing Carter's problem.

At that point, the family did begin intensive counseling, and the 17-year-old was put in a treatment program. They made sure that Carter never had to be alone with him again, or even be in the same house.

In her compelling book, *I Know Why the Caged Bird Sings*, Maya Angelou writes about her elective mutism after a childhood rape by her mother's boyfriend. She had experienced a very traumatic courtroom interrogation and after the trial, the man who had raped her was killed before he could serve his sentence. She suffered terrible guilt on top of the trauma of the sexual abuse. She says in the book:

> Just my breath carrying my words out might poison people and they'd curl up and die like the black fat slugs that only pretended.
>
> I had to stop talking.
>
> I discovered that to achieve perfect personal silence all I had to do was to attach myself leechlike to sound. I began to listen to everything. I probably hoped that after I had heard all the sounds, really heard them and packed them down, deep in my ears, the world would be quiet around me. I walked into rooms where people were laughing, their voices hitting the walls like stones, and I simply stood still – in the midst of the riot of sound. After a minute or two, silence would rush into the room from its hiding place because I had eaten up all the sounds.
>
> In the first weeks my family accepted my behavior as a post-rape, post-hospital affliction. (Neither the term nor the experience was mentioned in Grandmother's house, where Bailey and I were again staying.) They understood that I could talk to Bailey, but to no one else.
>
> Then came the last visit from the visiting nurse, and the doctor said I was healed. That meant that I should be back on the sidewalks

playing handball or enjoying the games I had been given when I was sick. When I refused to be the child they knew and accepted me to be, I was called impudent and my muteness, sullenness. For a while I was punished for being so uppity that I wouldn't speak; and then came the thrashings, given by any relative who felt himself offended.[29]

Eventually, a woman in the community took Maya, then called Marguerite, under her wing, brought her back to her house for special attention and read to her, encouraging her to read out loud to herself. In time, she was able to speak again.

Sometimes secrets are so enormous that children are afraid to talk because they might say them. It is important to teach children when it is the right time to keep a secret and when the secret should be told.

We saw another child, Bonnie, a first-grader who was wetting herself in school and was uncooperative with the teacher. She was a prime lesson in the dangers of class prejudice. On her visit to the DEC, both she and her father were dressed in stained clothing that was too small for their bulging bellies. The little girl's hair was dirty and hung in her face. She smelled of urine because she had had an accident that morning. I have to confess that we were expecting her to be in the borderline or delayed range, considerably behind her age, and made the assumption that she was wetting because she acted like a younger child in her overall behavior.

Were we in for a shock! Bonnie blew the top off of all our tests. Her IQ was 143. She was also friendly, polite, and liked to talk – a lot. She was altogether a delight to work with.

Bonnie told us that she was terribly bored and unhappy in school. The material was far too easy for her, and the teacher wouldn't let her read on her own or leave the group to work on her own. The children teased her for being overweight. We realized that she also wasn't changing her underpants regularly, and her parents hadn't thought to tell her to do so. Therefore, she smelled bad and the area around her urethra was often raw and irritated, which just made her feel more urgency to urinate.

I worked with her on the wetting problem through some hypnosis/ mental imagery over a period of time. I first showed her a picture of her urinary system, explaining how it worked and showing her where the muscles that held the urine in were. Then while she was in a relaxed and suggestible state, I talked about how muscles can learn, the way they learn to walk and jump and turn a somersault. We talked about her telling the muscles to stay shut until she was ready to go to the toilet.

She was very quick to make suggestions about ways that she could remember this, including having a fairy who kept the muscle shut with her magic wand. The more the child makes up his or her own imagery, the better this therapy technique works. Eventually, her daytime wetting improved, though she still sometimes wet at night.

Her father was overwhelmed and bursting with pride about her intelligence testing. He and his wife decided to sit down with the teacher and the principal to work out a program that was more appropriate for Bonnie. They were able to get an Individualized Educational Program (IEP) for her, which helped her behavior considerably. We also let the teacher know about the children's teasing so she could listen for it and stop it.

Of course, Bonnie had to take some responsibility, too. She had to agree to cooperate in school and to tell the teacher when something was bothering her. She also had to change her underwear at least daily and to keep an extra pair at school for when she wet herself.

Things did improve during the period of time I saw Bonnie, though her weight and sometimes her hygiene remained a problem. However, she was much happier with herself, and her parents had a new appreciation for her intelligence. She had formed a warm relationship with the teacher, who worked with her for an hour a day on more challenging projects. Though things were not perfect, life was looking up for her.

Kathy, our secretary, paged me through the intercom to my office.

"Terry just came in the door. He just walked right past. I think he's headed for your office."

"That's fine," I said, putting away my dictaphone. "I've got time."

Five seconds later, Terry came into my office, crying. His mother was only a few steps behind.

"Make it stop," he sobbed. "I can't think. I can't sleep. My mind keeps racing and racing and I feel like I'm going crazy."

This well-developed, muscular teenager, who looked about 16, was actually 12 and was holding onto his mother's hand. He put his head, with its thick, peroxide-blonde hair, on the sofa and moaned.

"It's okay, Terry," his mother and I soothed. "See if you can tell us what's upsetting you."

"I'm here to figure out how to help you," I added. "What's going on?"

"My thoughts," he said. "One moment I'm thinking about something and then my thoughts jump to something else and then they jump again, and I'm so worried all the time and then it makes me really scared and I feel like I've got to run around and I've got to do something! I've got to do something!"

"Okay, Terry," I said. "Take some deep breaths. Come on, breathe in and count to five slowly. Hold it for as long as you can. Then breathe out slowly. You can do it. Get control."

We had seen Terry a few days before. This eighth-grader's intelligence quotient tested at 158 – the brightest child we had ever tested. But Terry was having terrible problems. One moment he was despairing and almost suicidal. The next day, or even within the same day he was restless, active, had racing thoughts and talked non-stop. Sometimes he was wild and depressed at the same time. He had horrible insomnia. He frequently called his mother or father to stay up with him because he felt so out of control.

He had been seeing a psychologist, and we agreed with her that he needed to see a psychiatrist as quickly as possible. We all felt that he had rapid cycling bipolar illness. Instead of having up and down moods that lasted for several months before the cycle changed, he was having mood swings daily. But Medicaid had determined that it was not an emergency situation since he was not currently suicidal, and he was set up for an appointment with the doctor at the local mental health clinic in two weeks' time.

I am usually uncomfortable treating a serious psychological illness such as Terry had without the child first seeing a psychiatrist, but this was a real emergency. I had recently read an article about various medications that were best for adolescents with rapid-cycling manic-depressive illness and I put him on a starting dose of an anticonvulsant that was supposed to be helpful and began a mood-stabilizing drug. The psychologist was going to call and see if the psychiatrist could fit him in on an emergency basis.

Early in the evening, I got a call at home.

"Dr. Hays?"

"Yes?"

"Dr. Hays, it's Terry. I've got to talk to you. I can't take this medicine."

"Why not, Terry?"

"I researched it on the Internet. It says that the medicine can give you ataxia, tinnitus, headaches, stomach-aches, and severe rashes. How do I know that's not going to happen to me?"

Terry knew what all the medical words meant, no doubt about that.

"Terry, listen. We're going to keep a very careful eye on you. At the first sign of any side effects, you let your mom or dad know what's going on. Most people don't have those problems, and some of them are dose-related. Your regular doctor is going to be checking your blood levels regularly."

"But sometimes people have idiosyncratic reactions to these things!"

"That's very rare. But I promise you, Terry, we're going to keep an eye on all that. It's good to know a lot about your illness. But you are 12 years old. That's what your parents and I and Mickey [the psychologist] are here for – to take care of you and do the worrying. What we want you to do is stop worrying and turn it over to us. You've spent enough time eating yourself up inside."

"My reading indicates that rapid-cycling bipolar illness is one of the most difficult types to treat and that the prognosis is not good. What will this mean for when I'm an adult, Dr. Hays?"

"You don't need to get worried about that now, Terry. Really. You need to take one day at a time. Now listen to some soothing music and get some sleep. If you absolutely have to, take a sleeping pill."

"Dr. Hays?"

"Yes?"

"Sometimes being smart isn't such a great thing, huh?"

"No, it isn't. I know what you mean. I promise you that we'll take care of you. You need to be the patient and let us pick up the responsible adult role. Now you get some rest and let me talk to your mom."

"Okay. Mo-meeeee! Phone."

I could hear her coming to the phone.

"Terry, honey, you forgot to do the dishes."

"Oh, Mom, do I have to? Why doesn't Marion do it?"

"She's got homework."

"She's always got homework. Marion gets all the breaks! It's not fair, Mom!" Then, in an aside to his sister, "Marion – Mom says you have to do the dishes!"

"Terry!"

Terry had gone back to being his normal 12-year-old self. It was baffling to see the 12-year-old childishness coupled with the adult mentality. It must have been confusing for Terry, too.

Today, Terry is by no means over the hump. He is going to be struggling with his disease and his intelligence for some time to come. I only hope that his intelligence will help him find ways to cope with his disease. But it might cause him to become more obsessive, as his sponge-like mind absorbs more and more information about bipolar illness, about medications, and about problems that can arise during his treatment.

Being so smart will also make him lonely until he finds other people of similar intelligence. Only 1 percent of the population has an IQ of over 140 and, although I certainly do not think IQ is by any means the only measurement of intelligence nor a guarantee of getting along in life, it does influence the things that people find interesting and the companions they enjoy.

Being gifted is definitely a mixed blessing, though most of us know that being different from the crowd in any way gets easier as one gets older. I go to a "nerd" party given annually by friends. Once a year all the guests dress up as intellectually-adept-but-socially-inept people in various guises: at a prom, celebrating the millennium (2001, of course), or participating in the Olympics (with a floppy discus and a math triathlon). The reason we find this so funny is because all of us who go to these parties were ourselves nerds in high school. Some of us may have had a measure of popularity, but we all had to hide the fact that we were goal-oriented and smart, that our interests were unusual by high-school standards, and that we found some of what the in-crowd did immature and boring.

So it's fun to play the part with total abandon, something we would never have dared to do in high school, because as adults we are all relatively successful and happy, and can look back on our former selves with affectionate laughter.

Chapter 20

School

She took my hand and squeezed it. "You sold yourself short.
You could've been more than a teacher and a coach."
    I returned the squeeze and said, "Listen to me, Savannah.
There's no word in the language I revere more than the word *teacher*.
My heart sings when a kid refers to me as his teacher and it always
has. I've honored myself and the entire family of man by becoming
one."

Pat Conroy, The Prince of Tides

I remember my good teachers vividly even now. My third-grade teacher,
Mrs. Schoen, read to us every day: *Johnny Tremain, North to Freedom*, and
other books I have read many times since.[30] We all sat enthralled, leaning
forward over the tops of our desks to catch every word. She also taught us
songs from different countries, which I have taught my own children.

It was also a teacher who, in a roundabout way, started my interest in
science. I had always been more humanities oriented, preferring my
English, writing, art, and music classes. Then, in between seventh and
eighth grade, horror of all horrors, our English teacher gave us a required
summer reading list. One of the books was *Great Science Fiction Stories*, edited
by a librarian named Cordelia Titcomb Smith.[31] I dreaded reading it,
imaging Buck Rogers and "shoot-'em-up-with-space-lasers" stories. Late in
August, with school looming in the near future, I started it.

I devoured it. It made me realize that science could spur the imagination,
that it could take a fact and begin to ask "what if?" There was a story about a
boy who turned out to be an extraordinary genius because his parents had

been exposed to radiation. Another was about an anarchist who tried to infect a country with cholera bacteria; yet another about aliens with unusual powers who had accidentally crashed their spaceships on Earth and had to adapt.

Then in high school, I fortunately had a series of excellent teachers who continued to spur my interest in the sciences. My biology teacher took us to the ocean to collect marine biology specimens to study and my physics teacher had us to his house to see Comet Kohoutek with his telescope. They went out of their way to make science come alive.

In my opinion, next to parents, there is no one more influential on one's life than an inspiring teacher.

There are still wonderful teachers, and they don't get anything like the respect they deserve. I don't think anyone who isn't very familiar with the current school system can understand what teachers have to do nowadays. The changes that have occurred in education and educational philosophy since the late 1970s have made a good education accessible to a much larger sector of the population. However, having a much more heterogeneous group of pupils makes a teacher's job much, much more difficult.

Imagine a typical third grade now. Ms. Parker is at one of the groupings of desks, working with some children who are having trouble understanding something. Other children are working diligently on their own. One boy is rocking his desk back and forth, and the bumping on the floor is very distracting to everyone around him. She asks him to please stop rocking. He stops for a moment and then starts drumming on his desk. He is not getting his work done. His mother forgot to give him his medicine for his ADHD that morning.

Another child, a girl in a wheelchair, is working at a computer on the side.

"Ms. Parker, I can't get the program to work."

"Work on your own for a moment, boys and girls." Ms. Parker goes over to help.

There is a knock at the door.

"Yes?"

"I've come to get Amanda for speech class."

"Okay, Amanda, gather up your books. You can finish the work when you get back."

Amanda goes out. The children watch her.

Ms. Parker glances at the clock.

"Miguel, Tasha, and Tiffany – it's time for you to go to see Mr. Miyomi for resource class [special learning specifically geared to the child's problems]."

They leave. A child comes back in from occupational therapy.

"Ia, we were working in our math books."

Ia gives her a puzzled look.

"Pao, will you show Ia where we are in the book, please?"

Pao translates into Hmong.

"Boys and girls, finish up your math and put it away. Then get out your English books, please."

"Ms. Parker, will you read to us some more from that book – the one about the kids who hide in the museum?"

"Oh yeah, please, please," come pleas from all over the class.

"I will if we have time. Right now we have to look over our nouns, verbs, and adjectives. That's going to be on the end of the year test."

There are groans. The boy whose mother forgot his medication is poking another boy in the back with his pencil.

"Cut it out, jerk!"

"Boys! Robert, please pull a card. One more card, Robert, and you'll have to stay after school. Trey, name-calling is not acceptable. Apologize to Robert."

Another face appears at the door.

"Ms. Parker, telephone call for you."

Okay, maybe that would be a particularly hectic day. But it's not that far-fetched. I have been to schools to meet with teachers and observe patients, and I've seen these scenarios. Teachers deserve our undying admiration. The vast majority of them have to wear an enormous number of hats and are still dedicated to their jobs. Yet because their pay is low, many of the best leave education to find work that pays better and provides more positive feedback than they receive in the classroom.

Of course, in many ways, Ms. Parker's third grade as it was just described is an ideal classroom. The school and the teacher are trying to give each child exactly what he or she needs. Children of different ethnic and religious groups are being schooled together. Children are learning that their classmates have all sorts of special needs and that children with disabilities are a lot like them. Such heterogeneity works especially well when children with severe learning difficulties or behavior problems are able to work one-on-one with an aide.

However, classes like these also have problems. Lack of sufficient funding to meet all these needs sometimes makes the ideal less feasible, and so children who are mainstreamed sometimes find themselves swimming upstream without assistance. Children without learning difficulties do not always have their full needs met because another child is disruptive or demands a lot of extra attention from the teacher. Children who are slow but not actually learning disabled in the official sense of the phrase do not receive extra help (more about that later).

There is a wonderful documentary about a class that successfully includes a child with Down syndrome called *Educating Peter.*[32] It is a tribute to mainstreaming children in regular classrooms. What is notable is that Peter's teacher is very enthusiastic about working with him, there is loads of parental support, and the principal is very aware of what's going on in the classroom. When problems arise with Peter's behavior, there is a psychologist who comes to talk to all the classroom children and suggest how they handle Peter. The experiment is a tremendous success. And in that situation, I'm sure it would be. However, that kind of background support is rarely available.

"Inclusion," or mainstreaming, is the catchword of the early twenty-first century. In most cases, I think it's great. But I do feel that it should not be done unless sufficient resources are available to see that the mainstreamed child's needs are met. I also think that it is a decision that should be revisited regularly looking at the advantages and disadvantages to the disabled child and to his or her classmates. North Carolina kindergartens, for example, usually include a number of children who are developmentally delayed, and they often have to sink or swim. If they're sinking, they can have a lot of behavior problems. Kindergarten classes have an assistant teacher, but they are also frequently twice the size of other grades. The teachers have their hands full.

I have visited classes where a child in this situation was completely lost and had no friends. I have also seen classrooms where the teacher was beside herself because she ended up having to give so much time to a child with special problems that she had no time for the other kids. In some cases, a child who communicates poorly is aggressive to the others because she cannot express her feelings. I have to confess that if I were a parent with an "able" child in this type of situation, I would resent it, particularly if the aggressive child was hurting mine.

I have a few other gripes with the approach of the North Carolina public schools to their special-needs children (and with that of many other states as well). One is the lack of help for children who have borderline IQs – IQs between 70 and 80. These children are not mentally retarded. They would qualify for help if they were. They are not classified as learning disabled by the definition previously mentioned in this book: the 15-point discrepancy between IQ and an area of academic achievement. Yet they are less capable, at least in verbal and logical-mathematical skills (those that schools expect their students to master) than 95 percent of the population.

I have been involved in situations time and time again where children are achieving academically at a level "commensurate with their IQ." In other words, a fifth grader may be reasoning and thinking at a late third-grade level, and his reading level is also at late third grade. This would not be considered underachievement for his so-called potential, so it means that he doesn't (officially) need help Yet he is in the fifth grade and is expected to be working at approximately a fifth-grade level.

Aren't these, I ask myself, exactly the children who would benefit most from academic assistance? In terms of their future adaptability in society and their productivity as wage-earners, aren't they more likely to profit from help than a child who is, say, severely or profoundly developmentally delayed? It doesn't seem fair. We at the DEC know something is wrong with the system when we heave a sigh of relief that a child who had previously had an IQ of 72 has a repeat IQ of 69. It doesn't really indicate any difference (except statistical variation) in his or her intelligence, but the second measurement will open up a world of resources for the child. Clearly, more services are needed for these children.

All this brings up the question of how society wants to spend its money. At the moment, most school systems do not give physical therapy to children who might need it if their physical problem is not interfering with their "school function." That means that a child with spastic diplegia (cerebral palsy affecting only the legs) who can get around the school, get up the stairs in time to get to class, and carry a tray and eat lunch without difficulty will not receive physical therapy – that is, unless the child's parents want to pay for it privately. I understand the school's reasoning. After all, the line has to be drawn somewhere. Except that the child's family may not have health insurance or Medicaid and may not be able to afford private therapy. It is hard to know what the right answer is.

If I were absolute monarch of the country (president is nowhere near powerful enough!), basic health care would be free. I would have compulsory childcare classes for middle-school boys and girls, offer some sort of tax incentive to families whose adolescents choose to spend a year before college doing volunteer work for schools or other social programs, and make job-shadowing with work experience a far more frequent part of the public-school program in high school, especially for those teens who are not college-bound.

And I would cut way back on compulsory testing, the dreaded end-of-grade finals (EOGs) looming over the children until the end of school. At least I would make them far less important as a measure of performance.

I do think there is a standard to which children should be held and I, too, think that the 3 Rs are important. To me, though, the specter of the end-of-grade testing looms far too threateningly throughout the year, strongly influencing the way that children are taught. I suspect that most teachers would agree with me.

What happens when you create a test; tell students, teachers, and administrators that it is the most important measurement of achievement for all of them; and then inform the adults that their salaries and monies given to their schools will depend on its results?

It's pretty obvious that almost everything the teacher does all year will be geared to the test. In many cases that means no field trips, far fewer digressions on related topics that may be interesting but not on the test, and less time for explanations ("Sorry, we don't have time to go into that – we have to cover what's going to be on the test.") Don't believe it? Ask any teacher.

Bob Chase, the president of the National Education Association, says the following:

As a matter of fairness and accuracy, no student should be judged based on one test, given on one day, once a year. Any test should be just one component of a multifaceted approach to assessing a child's – or a school's – progress… Teachers are passionate on this issue. We are deeply concerned that tests are swallowing America's schools – and spitting out a diminished educational experience.

In a growing number of states, it seems as though the tests are driving everything. They are driving promotion and graduation decisions. They are driving – and distorting – the entire classroom experience of teachers and students. And they are driving many of our most skilled and creative teachers to look for other careers.[33]

Once a week for about three months before the end-of-grade tests, my son's middle school devoted one day to reviewing only English and Math, the two areas that would be tested. Everyone participated, whether they needed the review or not. On those days, my son did not get Science and Social Studies, his two favorite subjects. It did not seem to matter that the class didn't get through the Science and Social Studies books by the end of the year.

The traditional eighth-grade field trip to the Outer Banks, which introduced the kids to sites significant to North Carolina's early history, was canceled in favor of giving the children who failed the test the first time an opportunity to review and take it again.

Before the test, there was a day-long pep rally where teachers and administrators supposedly built up the students' confidence by having a "You can do it! Do it for the school!" message in the gym and giving out End-Of-Grade T-shirts.

In ninth-grade English, the kids reviewed grammar, vocabulary, and definitions of poetic terms but wrote no essays. When I asked why, the teacher told me that she would like to assign essays, but that the other information was what the end-of-grade test for ninth grade required. So there was no time for essays. Eventually, she did give a few writing assignments, because I urged the curriculum director to add on this requirement. In no way was this omission the teacher's fault. She had been given an order about what to teach in her class.

A friend of my daughter's, and a very able student, took an end-of-class test in American History on a day that she felt ill. She knew she had done very poorly and had even left a number of the essays blank. The assistant principal was angry with her because he said that her score on the test, especially from such a bright student, would "make the school look bad."

It's hard to imagine the level of anxiety that is caused by the push for good scores on these tests. It is bad enough for a regular student, but for a child with learning disabilities or one that is not academically able, the tests are a nightmare. Children bite their nails to the quick, burst into tears at nothing, and have trouble sleeping. And the US government is proposing to increase the frequency of these exams to the point where first-graders may be required to take them.

Sometimes the school will agree to give a special-needs child extra time on the test or to let a child with a learning disability have the test orally. This is certainly helpful for those children who know the material but cannot always indicate what they know in a standard testing situation. And I do not feel that this is preferential treatment. One wouldn't expect a child who was blind to take a test that she was required to read, unless it were in Braille.

The documentary *How Difficult Can This Be?* is a great eye-opener for someone who cannot understand what it is like to have a learning disability.[34] The narrator puts people without learning disabilities into situations where they are incapable of responding correctly because of ignorance, stress, high-speed talking, difficulty of the material and even ridicule. I recommend it to any teacher or parent who has a child with learning difficulties.

Chapter 21

Bullying

"What's your second name, Francis?" said Miss Wade.

"Chegwidden," said Francis, using the pronunciation as it had been taught.

Miss Wade, kindly but puzzled, said, "Did you say Chicken, Francis?"

"Cheggin," said Francis, much too low to be heard above the roar of the thirty others, who began to shout, "Chicken, Chicken!" in delight. This was something they could get their teeth into. The kid in the funny suit was called Chicken! Oh, this was rich!...
The boys decided that it was great fun to harry Francis across the line (to the girls' part of the playground) because anybody called Chicken was probably a girl anyway...

Teachers patrolled both playgrounds, carrying a bell by its clapper, and usually intent on studying the sky. Ostensibly guardians of order, they were like policemen in their avoidance of anything short of arson or murder. Questioned, they would probably have said that the Cornish child seemed to be popular; he was always in the centre of some game or other.

Robertson Davies, What's Bred in the Bone

The school shootings in the United States have made everyone aware of what horrible repercussions ridicule and bullying can have. Although, obviously, many factors led these emotionally troubled students to shoot their peers, one similarity between all the cases has been the alienation these children felt because of the way they were treated by their peers, and sometimes even by teachers, at school.

In the Internet discussions that Americans had about these shootings, many people wrote in to say that they, also, had been bullied and brutalized by their peers for being different in some way. Many of them expressed the helplessness and the rage that they had felt. The message that was conveyed by so many was, "I wanted to hurt them. I had fantasies of killing them. However, I didn't because I knew it was wrong. If it hadn't been for…[a parent, a teacher, a coach, a counselor, a best friend] to help me through this difficult time, I might have taken the same path as these kids."

It seems clear that if children have no support system and if no adult is vigilantly supervising their behavior, children are at much higher risk of acting out their hatred. Or they may turn their hatred inward. Yearly, at least ten children or teens kill themselves as a direct result of school bullying.

Bullying must be stopped. Just as there is a zero-tolerance for weapons such as knives and guns, there should be the same policy for bullying. I am not of the school of thought that believes "I don't care who started it. Both of you are punished." On the contrary, it is important to know who started it and even to hear both points of view. I remember how much I resented it when an adult said those words, and I had not been the one at fault.

For not only are the children who are bullied in danger – the bullies themselves are headed for serious trouble in life. There has been a study done at the University of Bergen in Norway that indicated that of those children who are still bullying others by middle school, 60 percent end up in trouble with the law or in jail as adults. Bullying, in this study, included physical and verbal abuse of other children.[35]

I have seen an example of this myself. There was a child in a class where I used to teach Spanish once a week who was a bully in the way that girls can be. She was only mildly physically aggressive, but she was severely verbally abusive. She would choose a particular girl to ostracize for a while and make her life miserable. Then she would arbitrarily move on to another girl. The other girls frequently would go along with her even though they might be the next target. Unfortunately, bullies can be quite popular. They are not necessarily disliked for their behavior, but rather admired. And feared.

A few months ago, I saw in the local newspaper that this girl, now 18, had been arrested for assault and battery. It does not surprise me, but it is sad. If her parents, her teachers, and the school had stopped the behavior and impressed upon the other students that cruelty like this would not be tolerated at all, it might have made a difference. I don't know.

Children who are bullies have generally not learned compassion. They simply do not understand how other people feel. They can be taught empathy, but it is increasingly difficult as they get older.

I suffered through a period of being bullied as a child, but fortunately, we moved and I did not have the problem at my new school. Still, I remember well the boy who used to sharpen his pencils (the two of us sat beside each other at the back of the class beside the pencil sharpener) and then poke the point into my arm. He also used to punch me, hard. The teacher did nothing to stop this behavior, despite my complaints and calls from my parents. In fact, when she rearranged the seating plan, she put us together again.

"Boys tease girls to show them that they like them," she said. I wonder if this boy is now a man who abuses his wife.

One method that is used by many psychologists is meant specifically to instill compassion and an understanding of other's feelings. It is a method that I often recommend to parents.

When the child is aggressive to another person, he is sharply rebuked with the reminder that "Hitting hurts. It is not acceptable." Then he is thoroughly ignored while all attention is given to the victim. The victim and the bully are then brought together.

"Tell him how you feel," the adult tells the victim. If the victim is a very small child, they probably need to be helped with this by the adult.

"You really hurt me. It makes me mad at you. I don't want to play with you right now," the victim might say.

The aggressor is asked to repeat what the victim said. "He said that I hurt him and he's mad at me."

Then the victim is asked what the aggressor can do to make him feel better. Depending on the age of the child, this may vary. A small child might suggest a hug or sharing a toy. An older child might suggest that the bully carry his lunch tray, bring her a flower, take over a chore for a few days. The suggestion should not be humiliating to the aggressor. If it is a chore that can be repeated over several days, it gives the child multiple reminders that doing something kind for another person can be rewarding and is a way of apologizing.

Other methods I have found helpful in controlling childhood bullying include encouraging bullies to keep a journal and write or draw out their feelings of anger, teaching them how to verbalize their anger, and stopping the aggression before it occurs by interfering verbally.

An adult might say, "Uh-oh. I see Ricky raising the stick to hit Molly. It looks like someone's about to get hurt. Quick! Get away from each other and think about this before you do anything." The children may need to be separated physically if the situation is too volatile.

A much more controversial subject is the use of spanking for discipline. The American Academy of Pediatrics has issued a statement that discourages spanking because, first, it is not very effective in preventing a behavior on a long-term basis; second, it teaches that hitting is okay if one person is bigger; and third, children who have been repeatedly spanked are more likely to be aggressive when they are older.[36]

A study at the Family Research lab at the University of New Hampshire that asked parents about their disciplinary practices indicated that 90 percent of US parents use corporal punishment; 25 percent of parents start spanking when their child is six months old and half spank their child by 12 months; 42 percent reported they had spanked their child sometime in the week before the survey.

A few studies have also shown that children who are regularly spanked have more academic problems and are less likely to finish college. They are also more prone to drug and alcohol use, depression, and anxiety.[37] It should be noted, however, that the spanking may not have caused these problems.

I think the main reason why all this is so controversial is that most of today's adults were spanked as children, and they feel as if they turned out fine. Most of them probably did. However, Americans are a pretty violent nation, and it's not just because of the easy access to guns, though I think that is a factor in the number of people who get seriously hurt. (After all, Lizzie Borden had an axe, not a gun, and killed only two people instead of twenty.) But violence is all around us. Look at road rage, fistfights, drive-by shootings, child abuse, and domestic violence, especially compared to other nations.

When my family was in Switzerland, where all men serve in the military and are required to be able to shoot well, we saw men on their way to target practice walking nonchalantly down the street or getting onto a bus carrying a semi-automatic rifle. No one blinked an eye; this was simply not dangerous in such a nonviolent culture.

It is also interesting that in some countries, like Sweden and Japan, spanking is simply not considered an acceptable form of punishment for children. Swedish and Japanese children are certainly well-behaved, so spanking is apparently not a requirement for good behavior.

In case all this sounds nauseatingly politically correct, I should qualify these statements by commenting that, personally, I don't think spanking children very *occasionally* damages them for life. It's the use of spanking as a systematic and frequent form of discipline that I strongly object to.

Dr. Alvin Poussaint of Harvard University points out that "fear of getting caught doing the wrong thing is very different from learning to behave because it is the right thing to do."[38] The use of spanking on a regular basis as a means of punishing a child – as opposed to using methods of discipline that involve explaining why a behavior is inappropriate – may keep children from developing an understanding of a higher morality.

Chapter 22

The Unkindest Cut: Terminal Illness

Crib Death

The rocker's creak inexorably sounds
In that still, forsaken room,
Its desolate technology
Mocking the Marrimeko children
Poised prancing on the wall:
The IV pole, now a barren, silver needle;
The heavy bulk
Of the respirator,
No longer groaning its weary sigh;
The curtain, halfway drawn,
A futile tribute to her private grief;
Every detail of her personal holocaust
Stamped on her face
As indelibly
As an Auschwitz tattoo.
The nurses have finally left her,
Taking with them the small body
She cradled in cramped arms.
And now she rock and rocks,
Beginning her lonely journey,
Her fingers twisted across her face
Like tangled vines.

Written about an experience that occurred
while working in the Emergency Room

The hardest job of all for a pediatrician is telling parents that their child has a terminal illness. I don't have to do it often, but we do sometimes see a child who we discover is much more ill than was originally suspected.

Three-year-old Bernie's mother was concerned about his development, but she was even more concerned about his walking. He had been walking fine, she said, until he broke his leg. He had been climbing on the monkey bars when he slipped and fell, bringing his shinbone sharply into contact with the metal bar.

He went to the hospital where an orthopedist put a cast on his leg, and they began the usual process of waiting for the bone to heal. While in a cast, Bernie was carried a lot by his parents, and he also maneuvered himself on his crutches. After the cast was removed, Bernie could not walk. His mother called the orthopedist, who was puzzled, but said that maybe he just had to get some practice again. He repeated an X-ray and indicated that the break was fully healed.

"He'll just get up one of these days and walk again," he said. "Have him try to bear weight while holding onto furniture and walk that way for a while."

Bernie could do that but a month passed, and he still couldn't walk more than a few steps without falling. He crawled or scooted on his bottom to get around. "He was a late walker," said his mother. "He didn't walk until 16 months. Actually, for a long time he walked everywhere on his knees. It was really funny. Then he finally got up, and then he was everywhere and into everything. So I never worried about it."

Bernie was a very cute boy with shaggy red-brown hair, a mischievous smile, and freckles everywhere. He cooperated well with all the testing and seemed to enjoy being at the DEC. His exam was normal except for some mild tightness around the ankles, and big calves.

"Let's see you get up from the floor, Bernie," I said.

Bernie gave us his big grin and set all his attention on getting up from his sitting position on the floor. First he got to a crawling position. Then to a kneel. Slowly, he got on one foot in a half-crouch. As he straightened up to a stand, he grabbed just above his knees with each hand and pushed on his legs to straighten them.

Lela and I looked at each other. Uh-oh. A Gower's sign. A Gower's sign, I have learned, is something never to be ignored. It is this classic way of getting off the floor when one's quadriceps, the front thigh muscles, are very weak. It is one of the first signs of muscular dystrophy.

"Did Bernie ever show any signs of muscle weakness before he broke his leg?" I asked.

"No, I don't think so," she said. "The only thing I remember is that about six months ago, he would wake up in the night sometimes and say that his legs hurt. Our doctor said it was growing pains. We would massage it and it would go away."

Lela and I felt Bernie's calves again. They were definitely large and they felt firm. We knew that in muscular dystrophy, the calves enlarge, not because they are well muscled, but because fat infiltrates the tissue.

Bernie laughed. "Tickles!" he said, squirming away.

When we sat down with Bernie's parents, we went over his test scores. In general, Bernie's intelligence and language scores were in the low average range, meaning that he was functioning at an age level of two-and-a-half in areas that do not involve movement. This is not a delay, but a child with low average abilities may have difficulty at school.

But, as I explained, I did wonder if his inability to walk had to do with an underlying weakness that had worsened during the period of time that Bernie was not using his muscles. I wanted to order a blood test, a creatinine phosphokinase (CPK), to see if there were any signs of muscle damage.

There was no point in explaining further at that point unless the parents had asked specifically what we were looking for. After all, we might be wrong. They didn't ask.

I got the blood test results back a few days later. An abnormal CPK is usually still well under one hundred. This CPK was 25,000. I suddenly had a headache and had to sit down. There was no question that Bernie had muscular dystrophy. He had probably been just barely making it on what muscle he had to walk and run and climb, and when he was in the cast, the normal atrophy of the muscle that occurs with disuse had seriously worsened the problem. He didn't bounce back, the way most children would have done.

I drove to the parents' house in a nearby county to give them the news. They were expecting something bad. I had told the mother I was coming out and I had also said that it was important that both parents be there.

How do you say to a family, "Your son has a terrible muscle disease. It's incurable. He's going to get weaker and weaker until his muscles finally can't even support his breathing. He won't live through his teens."

Of course, you don't say that. At least not all in the first meeting. I told them that Bernie had muscular dystrophy and explained what it was and how the children who have it get very weak. I set them up to see the doctors and therapists at the Muscular Dystrophy Clinic in Charlotte for further tests, further advice, and to see what kind of muscular dystrophy Bernie had, though it was most likely Duchenne's. I also set them up with a geneticist. The problem is passed through the mother to her boys if they happen to get her bad carrier X chromosome with the defective gene; 50 percent of boys born to a carrier mother have the disease.

They cried. I cried. They didn't ask a lot of questions. If they had, I would have answered them. I believe people need to know the truth. On the other hand, parents often indicate when they can handle the truth, and it's usually only bit by bit and not right away.

Sometimes, a parent will want to know the worst case scenario right away. Recently, I saw a child whose IQ had dropped 20 points in a year and who was showing a severe tremor, some very unusual extraneous movements of the hands and tongue, and other unusual behaviors. I was quite worried that these were signs of some sort of deteriorating neurological disease.

I expressed my concerns to his parents and stated that he needed to see a neurologist as soon as possible. His mother listened intently.

"What is the very worst that could happen?" she asked. "Could he die?" Her eyes were dry, but I saw a mother who was hanging onto my every word, ready to spring into action like a tiger fighting for its cub's life.

"If these are signs of some type of neurological disease, it is possible that we can stop its progression. However," I took a deep breath, "yes, if it is one of the types that is incurable, he could conceivably die."

"I want to do every test we can possibly do – now," she said. "Yesterday, if possible."

She had snapped into "go" mode faster than most parents. For her, action was the best way to cope.

We recently had parents who had reacted little to the bad news that their daughter might have a degenerative ataxia (balance problem) although they nodded and said that they understood. They had no questions. As we always do, we encouraged them to call anytime or come back if they needed to. They left and they were back in an hour. Apparently they had gone home to tell a grandparent what had happened and realized they had no idea what we had said, except that it was very bad. That's what shock is all about. I suspect that it is nature's way of protecting us from overwhelming emotion we cannot handle all at once.

Because of this, I commonly say, "Now, it is very likely that you're going to go home and realize that you didn't take in everything that I said. That's okay. Please make a list of all the questions you have and come back when you need to."

We give parents handouts when it is appropriate and they always get a copy of the full report in a week or two. I can only hope that they appreciate being armed with information for the battle ahead.

For many parents, their religion is a resource from which they can draw great comfort and strength. Their knowledge that God is looking out for them and that there is a greater plan helps them to accept the tragedy of a seriously ill child. For others, a tragedy flings them into direct conflict with their beliefs: if God loves me, why did he cause this to happen? Is God punishing me? Grief can shake their beliefs to the core.

Each family has to cope in its own way. Acceptance comes gradually and may take many years for some. No one can know how he or she would react until put into the situation.

I have had the experience of seeing children who have accepted their terminal illness faster than their parents have. I will never forget a little girl of eight I took care of years ago in Minnesota. She had a rare type of leukemia and had received a bone-marrow transplant in the earlier days of this procedure. She was doing very poorly. Her immune system was not bouncing back and her blood counts weren't, either. We had little hope for her recovery.

Late one night, when I was giving her some pain medication and helping her put viscous lidocaine, another painkiller, on the sores in her mouth, she looked up and grabbed my hand.

"Tell me, Dr. Natasha, am I going to die?" She looked me square in the eyes.

"Dedra, I don't know. You are very sick, sweetheart."

"I'm dying," she told me. "I know I am."

I said nothing, just held her hand.

"Do you think you could tell my Mommy?" she said. "I don't think she knows it. She keeps talking about when we get home. I don't think I'm going home."

I couldn't speak, but I nodded. Dedra smiled and settled back in bed.

"I think I'll feel better if Mommy knows," she said. "But I don't want to tell her. I think I'll try to go back to sleep now."

She closed her eyes.

I quickly left the room, went to the nurses' station, and sobbed. It was just too much for me. Doctors need outlets, too, or they burn out. It is not always appropriate or expedient to show emotion on the job, at least not in many situations. You can't panic and cry during an emergency; it interferes with your work.

I think it is the reason that both my husband and I cry very easily in sentimental movies. It's a safe place. I know a child psychiatrist that works with terminally ill children who loves opera. She told me she goes to the opera and sobs her heart out.

As I said to the medical student I mentioned earlier who cried, if we stop caring, we lose what made us want to be doctors in the first place. Anyone can be a diagnostician given the education and the intelligence. It's compassion that keeps the connection between the doctor and the patient. You need both to be a truly good doctor.

I think that the majority of the DEC patients and their parents feel that we care about them. I am fortunate to work with a group of people who are dedicated to their jobs and consider it something of a mission to make life better for children.

Chapter 23

Ariel and Alex

My long-limbed, dancing insect girl
You shed transparent skins outgrown
Your tender arms and legs unfurl,
Still fragile, glistening wisps. Alone
You skitter on your way, to face
The taunting beaks of birds, the gust
Of sudden wind, fierce rain. This place
Is wild and perilous. Entrust
You to its wounds? I have no choice.
But once, I was your shelter. I
Could wrap you womb-warm in my arms
And scatter demons, hush your cry,
My kiss an amulet from harms
So easily dissolved. No more.
The enemies that would devour
You leave me paralyzed, my store
Of magic gone, my only power
A soothing, sympathetic voice.
But when your tender skin grows firm,
As it inevitably will,
May its resilience still affirm
That lingering vestige of my skill,
And may your courage but enhance
The spirit pulsing though your dance.

I can't write about so many children who have been important to me and not write about my own children, Ariel and Alex. For better or worse, I combined being a parent with doctoring from the very beginning, becoming pregnant in my internship with Ariel and, in my first year of private practice, with Alex.

I can't say it had been pleasant being pregnant during my residency or my early years of practice. In residency, when we stood forever in the halls on rounds, presenting cases and discussing them, sometimes I'd suddenly grab a chair and plop down.

"Sorry," I'd say. "I'm going to faint if I don't sit down!"

A "Code Blue" would send me racing up four flights of stairs, holding my belly all the way, to arrive at the scene of the emergency, gasping and unable to speak. I still worry about all the massive rushes of adrenaline I gave my babies while they were in the womb. They must have been as stressed as I was!

Those days are long gone now except in memory. It's hard to know how I managed; I just did.

Ariel is now 20 and a student at Oberlin College, Ohio, my alma mater. When she was born, she didn't cry or yell. Phil and I and my parents got to hold her in the first few hours of her life before she went back to the newborn nursery to be cleaned off. All that time she looked out on her new world with a solemn and slightly puzzled look on her face. She was a quiet baby in the nursery and nursed well from the beginning, starting to sleep through the night very quickly.

She talked quite early but was on the late side of normal walking, taking her first steps at 13 months, but not really walking comfortably until a month later. She was very affectionate with family members and her babysitter, but painfully shy with others.

She loved to be read to and to have pictures in books pointed out so she could name them. When Ariel was 14 months old my sister came to visit and discovered that she could identify several letters of the alphabet. So Kim and I decided to teach them all to her, and she mastered them by 15 months without any problem. She knew her numbers up to ten by 16 months, began reading individual words at two, and was reading quite well by three or four. This was not because we taught her to read. She learned because she would want me to put my finger under the words as I read to her and she would watch, carefully, until she had mastered them. I would sometimes read a word incorrectly or skip one if I was tired, and she would point to the word and correct me.

Ariel also loved music. She would sing and dance quietly by herself for hours on end, even as late as elementary school. She would go to choir practice with me and to ballet performances as a tiny girl and sit entranced the whole time without any wiggling and squirming.

"All right, time for our warm-up," the director would say, at choir. She would get out of her chair and stand with everyone else, trying to reach the notes with her little voice. She took this all very seriously.

When she was four years old, we went to a fair and she heard someone announce that there was going to be a singing contest that visitors could enter. She tugged on my arm and announced that she wanted to be in it. I couldn't believe that my shy little girl wanted to perform in front of a crowd of strangers, but she was adamant. I entered her, she performed like a trooper, and she won. (Naturally, I think the cuteness factor helped a lot, since she was by far the youngest participant.) From then on she was hooked on the theater.

However, this same child who read and sang so confidently was vastly less confident with people, especially other children. When a bunch of children were all together yelling and running around and being rambunctious, Ariel would shrink back into a corner and hide.

She did better with one or two children that she knew well. But any amount of urging her to join in the fun was totally counterproductive.

Adults who had the opportunity to get to know her liked her and told me how mature she was for her age. But we knew this was true only in some ways. I remember going over to a friend's house to pick her up for a party. While she got ready, her child, exactly Ariel's age, eight, sat with Phil and me, whom she knew only a little, and showed us a coffee table book on gardens that was in the room, discussing her favorites with us. We both knew that such poised and friendly behavior was way beyond Ariel's capabilities.

Ariel never responded to peer pressure at all, which, although admirable in many ways, caused her some major problems at school. She dressed the way she wanted to dress, she showed little interest in talking clothes and about who was going with whom, and she didn't seem interested in many of the things that interested her peers. She didn't go to many parties, and she would read, hang out with the family, write poetry, or play her guitar. Still, she was lonely and became somewhat depressed because she couldn't seem to find people who shared her interests. Plus, because she was quiet and different, she was something of a target for bullies and unkind children all the way up through middle school.

About tenth grade, she began to find more people who appreciated her for who she was. She began spending time with an older boy whose friends took her in, and she found other people who enjoyed acting and science and others of her interests. By the time she was a high-school senior she was a fairly prominent figure in school, known for her acting and her various "foreign accents" which she regularly used when reading aloud in class (and once, on a dare, for a school speech). She was a runner on the track and cross-country teams and the only liberal in the Political Issues club. She was outspoken about things she believed in, which sometimes brought her into philosophical clashes with the high-school principal.

Now, at college, she feels much more at home. She is taking lots of neuroscience and writing classes. She does martial arts, belly dances, and is an active environmentalist. She still feels different from other people some of the time but much, much less so. She has plenty of friends. She continues to be quite close to Phil and me and her brother, Alex.

Alexander was born three years after Ariel. It was clear from the start, when he came out into the world, yelling, that this was a different child from our daughter. He didn't sleep through the night until he was about ten months old and fed somewhat erratically. This was hard on me, since I had assumed that he would sleep easily like Ariel. When I started back to work part-time when he was six months old, I was frequently functioning on only four or five hours of sleep.

Alex walked well before a year and, by 15 months, could vault out of his crib by placing a foot on the rail, hurling his body over, hanging from the rail on the other side and dropping down to the ground. This meant forays into the refrigerator and among the pots and pans. Fortunately, I seemed to have a mother's sixth sense about these things and was always just barely behind him to rescue him before the danger became too severe. Nevertheless, we practically owned stock in the Emergency Room due to visits for stitches, emptying his stomach of poisonous pokeweed, and other emergency treatment. I was often at my wit's end. Once I heard a tiny voice singing, "Happy Birthday to You," and ran downstairs, knowing that I would find what I did, which was two-year-old Alex lighting matches and dropping them on the carpet when they began to scorch his fingers. That earned him a visit to the local fire department and a stern lecture from a fireman.

The one time I took Alex to choir with me, he got hold of two erasers at the blackboard and clapped them together until the air was filled with chalk dust. That was the last time he came along.

Interestingly enough, despite this little whirlwind's wild ways, I don't remember worrying that he had ADHD. He never had any problem concentrating when he wanted to. He certainly could pull a parent's chain, though.

He was, and still is, a wickedly accurate mimic, and it was very amusing to see him as a toddler unconsciously imitating me: backing out a little riding car to go somewhere and saying, "Got my list, got the garbage for the dump, got my purse, uh-oh – forgot my keys!" Then, hitting himself on the head in exasperation, he'd sigh, open the "car" door, go get the imaginary keys, and start over again. He also likes quoting the lines from movies in the voice of the appropriate actor. However, unlike his sister, who loves to be on stage, he recites them only for his friends and family.

He did have his acting moments, if they coincided with a current interest of his. I had a friend visiting from out of town when Alex was about five years old. She says that their first meeting will remain indelibly printed in her mind. He came running down the stairs, naked except for his underwear, painted completely blue, with a broom handle for a spear, yelling, "I'm a Celt, I'm a Celt!"

Even as a small child, Alex developed what I called "passions." First it was Robin Hood. Then it was World War II. Then it was Legos. He was like a sponge, wanting to learn everything he possibly could about whatever he was interested in at that point. He also learned to channel his very high activity level into sports. Soccer is a passion, and he is on several different teams. Math is another favorite.

Although he is a very good student and a reader like Ariel, Alex has always expressed frustration about doing things the teacher's way. He has been in trouble more than once for refusing to follow the exact procedure in solving a math problem or writing an essay. He has very little patience with what he considers superfluous, to the point of being belligerent at times. It continues to be very hard for Phil and me to convince him that sometimes it's just easier to do things (including chores!) the way others want them done, even if one doesn't agree. He also enjoys arguing for the sake of the debate, no matter how small the topic.

Socially, he has had few difficulties. His mischievous sense of humor and basic friendliness have helped. So has his interest in sports and competitive games. However, he still needs a lot of time alone, and he prefers friends who share his desire to master a skill, such as chess or a computer game.

In some ways, Ariel and Alex are similar. Like their parents, they are both independent thinkers, enjoy travel and having new experiences, are very goal-oriented, hyper-perfectionist, self-critical, and far too driven to achieve. They both have a strong sense of justice and enjoy debating an idea. Like their father, they are reserved with people they have just met and are prone to internalize stress. Also like Phil, they are both good at mechanical things, which are a mystery to me. Like me, they are fond of animals and enjoy a good joke or prank. Nature or nurture? I have no idea. Physically, Alex looks much more like me. Ariel is a mix, but primarily takes after Phil and his side of the family.

I am enormously proud of them, but also very aware of their shortcomings.

Two children, not so far apart in age, from the same genetic soup, raised in the same family, taught the same basic values, and yet so different. I know that just about all families experience this in their offspring.

As the only blonde, blue-eyed person in a brunette family, I was often asked as a child if I was adopted. If I had known more, I could have replied, "No, I'm just a genetic recessive!" But, of course, it is not only outward physical features that can play genetic tricks. Though environment certainly plays a part of forming a child's character, I am fully convinced from my patients and my own children that the chromosomal deck of cards they are given to play with makes an enormous difference in the outcome of the game. Or to use another game metaphor, it's just a toss of the cosmic dice.

Studies of twins reared apart support this amazingly. Details about their lives show unbelievable similarities, such as their both walking into water backwards and giving their children the same names. They tend to be more similar to each other in interests and intelligence than to their adoptive families. A famous University of Minnesota study on identical twins reared apart showed some similarites between twins that were so astounding that it changes our ideas of how genetics can influence our personalities. A pair of twins, one raised in Texas, one in Wyoming, met and discovered that they were both firefighters, both had droopy moustaches and aviator glasses, and both had considered a career in forestry. Another pair found that both wore rubber bands on their wrists and both sneezed loudly in order to attract attention. Other similarities between these twins included having similar phobias such as fear of escalators.[39]

As for intelligence, the study showed an 86 percent correlation between identical twins raised together, a 60 percent correlation between fraternal twins raised together, and a 72 percent correlation between identical twins raised apart. This suggests that intelligence is multifactorial, but slightly more closely related to genetics.[40]

As parents, we often agonize, what could I have done differently? Where have I gone wrong? Is it my fault that Johnny has such a bad temper? If I had just spent more time playing with him, if I had just kept her out of daycare, if I had just…

I tend to fall into this trap as often as the next parent. But I think we need to remind ourselves that creatures of different genetic make-up respond differently to the same environmental stimulus. As well, we need to remind ourselves that we parents are only human and all we can do is to make the best decisions for our children that we know how to make at any one time, given the available information, our own shortcomings, and stresses.

Epilogue

Our hope for our children, no matter what their strengths and weaknesses, is for them to realize their potential and be happy adults who live fulfilling lives. I know that this is what I want for my children more than I want for them wealth, fame, or the other trappings of outward success.

Often parents look to me to be the guru who will tell them what to expect of their child's future. I am uncomfortable with the role of all-powerful seer into the future, and I explain to them that I do not have a crystal ball. However, we have to maintain belief in our children and in their capacity to adapt. We also have to adapt our way of viewing success. For example, when the father of a child with moderate to severe cerebral palsy asks me if his son will ever walk, I tell him that I do not know and ask him to think about what the important aspect of the question is. The important question is, really, "Will he be able to get around, to move from one place to another?"

"Change your feelings about the way you are asking about the goal and concentrate on accomplishing the goal in a different way," I might tell him. "If Stefan uses a crutch, a walker, or even a wheelchair, and he is able to go where he wants to go, then he is succeeding."

He is able to go where he wants to go. That says it all, doesn't it?

Alexander the Great and Julius Caesar had epilepsy. Alexander Graham Bell had a hearing loss. Louis Braille was blind. Theodore Roosevelt was a sickly child who had asthma and very poor vision. Stephen Hawking has amyotrophic lateralizing sclerosis (ALS). Itzhak Perlman has paralysis from polio. Beethoven became deaf at the height of his career. Mary Tyler Moore has diabetes. Winston Churchill and Woodrow Wilson both had learning disabilities. Sigmund Freud battled cocaine addiction and cancer. And that's only some of the famous people. The list goes on and on.

When loved ones have disabilities, obvious or hidden, we learn to take joy in the little successes. In every small increment of gain. And sometimes, we are even surprised with giant leaps of mankind.

Notes

1. Nickerson, H.J., Mathay, K.K., Seeger, R.C. *et al.* (2000) "Favorable Biology and Outcomes of Stage IV-s Neuroblastoma with Supportive Care or Minimal Therapy." *Journal of Clinical Oncology 18*, 3, 477–486.

2. McFate, K. (1995) *Making Welfare Work: Principles of Constructive Welfare Reform.* Washington, DC: Joint Center for Political and Economic Studies.

3. Glaser, D. (2000) "Child Abuse and Neglect and the Brain – A Review." *Journal of Psychology and Psychiatry 41*, 1, 97–116.

4. De Bellis, M.D. (2001) "Developmental Traumatology: the Psychobiological Development of Maltreated Children and its Implications for Research, Treatment, and Policy." *Development and Psychopathology 13*, 3, 539–564.

5. Jones, K.L. (1997) *Smith's Recognizable Patterns of Human Malformation*, 5th edn. Philadelphia, PA: W.B. Saunders, p.248.

6. Streissguth, A.P., Barr, H.M., Sampson, P.D., Bookstein, F.L. and Darby, B.L. (1989) "Neurobehavioral Effects of Prenatal Alcohol," Parts 1, 2, 3. *Neurotoxicology and Teratology 11*, 5, especially 493–507.

7. Frank, D., Augustyn, M., Grant Knight, W., Pell, T. and Zuckerman, B. (2001) "Growth, Development, and Behavior in Early Childhood Following Prenatal Cocaine Exposure." *Journal of the American Medical Association 285*, 1613–1625.

8. Morris, C.A., Demsey, S.A., Leonard, C.O., Dilts, C. and Blackburn. B.L. (1988) "Natural History of Williams Syndrome: Physical Characteristics." *Journal of Pediatrics 113*, 2, 316–326.

9. Semel, E. (1991) In R. Finn *Discover Magazine*, June, p.58.

10. Finucane, B., McConkie-Rosell, A. and Cronister, A. (1988) *Fragile X Syndrome: A Handbook for Families and Professionals.* Elwyn, PA: Ellwyn.

11. Zeschnigk, M. *et al.* (1997) "Imprinted Segments in the Human Genome." *Human Molecular Genetics 6*, 3, 387–395.

12. Koman, L.A., Mooney, J.F. and Smith, B.P. (1993) "The Use of Botulinum-A Toxin in the Management of Cerebral Palsy in Pediatric Patients." In B.R. Das Gupta (ed) *Botulinum and Tetanus Neurotoxins: Neurotransmission and Biomedical Aspects.* New York: Plenum Publishing Corporation, 518–587.

13. Sommerfelt, K., Markestad, T., Berg, K. and Saetesdal, I. (2001) "Therapeutic Electrical Stimulation in Cerebral Palsy: A Randomized, Controlled, Crossover Trial." *Developmental Medicine and Child Neurology 43*, 9, 609–613.

14. Dickman, C.A., Rekate, H.L., Shetter, A. and Sidell, A. (1988) "Posterior Rhizotomy for the Treatment of Spasticity." *BNI Quarterly 4*, 2, 20–23.

15. Stanley Greenspan, talk at Leo Croghan Conference, Raleigh, NC, 1999.

16. Fombonne, E. (1996) "Is the Prevalence of Autism Increasing?" *Journal of Autism and Development Disorders 26*, 6, 673–676.

17. Grandin, T. (1996) *Emergence: Labeled Autistic.* New York: Warner.

18.   Josephson, M. (1959) *Edison: A Biography*. New York: McGraw-Hill. p.16.

19.   Josephson, M. (1959) *Edison: A Biography*. New York: McGraw-Hill. p.100.

20.   Sacks, O. (1995) *An Anthropologist on Mars: Seven Paradoxical Tales*. New York: Knopf. p.xvi.

21.   Needleman, H. (2004) "Lead poisoning." *Annual Review of Medicine 55*, 209–222.

22.   Canger, R., Battino, D., Canevini, M.P., Fumarola, C. *et al.* (1999) "Malformations in offspring of women with epilepsy: a prospective study." *Epilepsia 40*, 9, 1231–6; Holmes, L.B., Harvey, E.A., Coull, B.A., Huntington, K.B., Khoshbin, S. *et al.* (2002) "The teratogenicity of anticonvulsant drugs." *New England Journal of Medicine 12*, 344, 15, 1132–8.

23.   Crawford, P. (2001) "CPD–Education and self-assessment: Epilepsy and pregnancy." *Seizure 10*, 3, 212–19.

24.   Bryk, M. and Siegel, P.T. (1998) "My Mother Caused my Illness: the Story of a Survivor of Munchausen by Proxy Syndrome." *Pediatrics 100*, 1, 1–7.

25.   Alan Guttmacher Institute (AGI) (1994) *Sex and America's Teenagers*. New York: AGI.

26.   Boyer, D. and Fine, D. (1992) "Sexual Abuse as a Factor in Adolescent Pregnancy and Child Maltreatment." *Family Planning Perspectives 24*, 1, 4–11, 19.

27.   Preliminary study at University of North Carolina, Chapel Hill, presented by Carol Shores, MD, Ph.D., 2000.

28.   Child Net Physician Network, Barton Schmidt.

29.   Angelou, M. (1970) *I Know Why the Caged Bird Sings*. New York: Random House Bantam Books, p.73.

30.   Forbes, E. (1945) *Johnny Tremain*. Boston, MA: Houghton Mifflin; Holm, A. (1965) *North to Freedom*. New York: Harcourt, Brace.

31.   Titcomb Smith, C. (1964) *Great Science Fiction Stories*. New York: Dell.

32.   Goodwin, T.C. and Wurzburg, G. (1992) *Educating Peter*. Video cassette from Films for the Humanities and Sciences.

33.   Chase, B. (2001) "Loudest Buzz of Rebellion Led by Engler." *Knight/Ridder Tribune*, July 21.

34.   Lavoie, R. (1974) *How Difficult Can this Be?* Peter Rosen Productions.

35.   Olweus, D. (1993) *Bullying at School: What We Know and What We Can Do*. Cambridge: Blackwell Publishing.

36.   American Academy of Pediatrics (AAP) (2000) "Policy Statement on Spanking." *Pediatrics 106*, 2, 343.

37.   Jackson, D.D. (1980) "Reunion of identical twins, raised apart, reveals some astonishing similarities." *Smithsonian 11*, 7, 48–56.

38.   Poussaint, A. (1999) "Spanking Strikes Out." FamilyEducation.com, September 27.

39.   *Newsweek*, November 8, 1993.

40.   Bouchard, T.J., Lykken, D.T., McGue, M., Segal, N.L. and Tellegen, A. (1990) "Sources of Human Psychological Differences: The Minnesota Study of Twins Reared Apart." *Science 250*, 223–228.

41.   Dennis, L. and Kunz, R. (1960) *The Story of Honey*. Canadian Beekeepers' Council (now Canadian Honey Council).

Appendix

I have always had a strong interest in bibliotherapy, the process of understanding and healing emotional problems through reading fiction related to the specific problem a person is having.

In thinking about this, I realized that one of my very favorite stories when I was very little was a book called *The Story of Honey*.[41] I think this is interesting because one of my first memories in life is of being stung by a bee and I had vivid nightmares about bees, some of which I still remember, until I was about three or four. *The Story of Honey* is all about how bees are good and help people. Now, my family keeps several hives and I am not scared in the least.

I do think children are often drawn to books that have meaning for them in a very personal way. In this appendix are books that cover some of the subjects that I have discussed in this book. They are meant both for children who have those problems and for adults, friends, and siblings who may need some more understanding of a child with special needs. Obviously, the list is incomplete, but these are books with which I am familiar, and which I recommend.

I have included some nonfiction in these listings, especially when there is not a lot of fiction on the subject available for children, but it is mainly fiction or autobiography. They include books for small children, school-age children, and young adults.

Since there are also many quality movies that cover these subjects, I have also listed a selection of these. Most are available on video or DVD.

Learning Disabilities
Bunting, E. (1990) *The Wednesday Surprise*. New York: Clarion.
Dahl, R. (1994) *The Vicar of Nibbleswicke*. London: Puffin.
DeClements, B. (1985) *Sixth Grade Can Really Kill You*. New York: Viking Kestrel.
Gehret, J.M.A. (1996) *The Don't-Give-Up Kid and Learning Differences*. Fairport, NY: Verbal Images.
Hansen, C. (1991) *Yellow Bird and Me*. New York: Clarion.
Levine, M.D. (1993) *All Kinds of Minds*. Cambridge, MA: Educator's Publishing Services.
Parish, P., *Amelia Bedelia* books, (numerous).
Peterseil, T. (1996) *The Safe Place*. New York: Pitspopany Press.
Polacco, P. (1998) *Thank You, Mr. Falker*. New York: Philomel.

Movie
How Difficult Can This Be?

Physical Disabilities (cerebral palsy, spina bifida, wheelchair-bound children, limb injuries, other)

Carlson, N. (1990) *Arnie and the New Kid.* New York: Viking.

Crutcher, C. (2003) *The Crazy Horse Electric Game.* New York: HarperTempest.

De Angeli, M. (1989) *The Door in the Wall.* New York: Doubleday.

Fassler, J. and Lasker, J. (1997) *Howie Helps Himself.* Chicago: Albert Whitman.

Forbes, E. (1943) *Johnny Tremaine.* Boston, MA: Houghton Mifflin.

Rabe, B. (1991) *Margaret's Moves.* New York: Dutton.

Voight, C. (1986) *Izzy Willy-Nilly.* New York: Atheneum.

Movies
The Big Chill
Coming Home
My Left Foot
Whose Life Is It, Anyway?

Malformations and Syndromes

Clarion, H. (1996) *Children with Facial Differences: A Parent's Guide.* Bethesda, MD: Woodbine House.

Hagenboon, M. (2001) *Living with Genetic Syndromes Associated with Intellectual Disabilities.* London: Jessica Kingsley Publishers.

Lucado, M. (2000) *You are Special.* Wheaton, IL: Crossway.

Philbrick, W.R. (1993) *Freak the Mighty.* New York: Blue Sky Press.

Movies
The Elephant Man
Mask
The Mighty
Roxanne
Simon Birch

Autism, Asperger syndrome

Faherty, C. (2000) *Asperger's: What Does it Mean to Me?* Arlington, TX: Future Horizons.

Hoopman, K. (2001) *Blue Bottle Mystery: An Asperger Adventure.* London: Jessica Kingsley Publishers.

Lears, L. (1998) *Ian's Walk: A Story about Autism.* Morton Grove, IL: Albert Whitman.

Rodowsky, C.F. (2001) *Clay.* New York: Farrar, Straus & Giroux.

Thompson, M. (1996) *Andy and His Yellow Frisbee.* Bethesda, MD: Woodbine House.

Movies
Family Pictures
Rain Man

Vision Impairments, Blindness
Little, J. (1991) *From Anna.* New York: HarperCollins.
Little, J. (1991) *Little by Little, A Writer's Education.* London: Puffin.
Vaughn, S. (1996) *Grandpa's Eyes.* Johnson City, TN: Overmountain Press.

Movies
Butterflies are Free
The Miracle Worker
Night Must Fall
A Patch of Blue
Wild Hearts Can't Be Broken

Hearing Impairments, Deafness
Butts, N. (1996) *Cheshire Moon.* Arden, NC: Front Street Press.
Kisor, H. (1991) *What's That Pig Outdoors?* New York: Penguin.
Lakin, P. (1994) *Dad and Me in the Morning.* Morton Grove, IL: Albert Whitman.
Millman, I. (1998) *Moses Goes to a Concert.* New York: Farrar, Straus & Giroux.

Movies
Children of a Lesser God
Cop Land
The Heart is a Lonely Hunter
Johnny Belinda
The Miracle Worker
Mr. Holland's Opus

Speech Problems
Lester, H. and Munsinger, L. (1999) *Hooway for Wodney Wat.* Boston, MA: Houghton Mifflin.
Sedaris, D. (2000) *Me Talk Pretty One Day.* Boston, MA: Little, Brown.

Movie
Nell

Mood Disorders, Depression, Bipolar Illness
Fuqua, J.S. (1999) *The Reappearance of Sam Webber.* Baltimore, MD: Bancroft Press.
Guest, J. (1982) *Ordinary People.* New York: Penguin.
Hamilton, D. and Owens, G. (1995) *Sad Days, Glad Days: A Story about Depression.* Morton Grove, IL: Albert Whitman.
Hawley, R.A. (1983) *The Headmasters' Papers.* Middelbury, VT: P.S. Eriksson.
Kulling, M. (1999) *Edgar Badger's Butterfly Day.* Greenvale, NY: Mondo.
Pipher, M.B. (1995) *Reviving Ophelia.* New York: Putnam.
Sullivan, F. (1997) *The Empress of One.* Minneapolis, MN: Milkweed.
Waltz, M. (2000) *Bipolar Disorders: A Guide to Helping Children and Adolescents.* Sebastopol, CA: O'Reilly.

Movies
(including movies about other mental illnesses)
Girl, Interrupted
One Flew Over the Cuckoo's Nest
Ordinary People

Obsessive Compulsive Disorder

Hesser, T.S. (1998) *Kissing Doorknobs*. New York: Delacorte.

Sedaris, D. (1999) *Naked*. Boston, MA: Little, Brown.

Tashjian, J. (1999) *Multiple Choice*. New York: Henry Holt.

Movie
As Good as It Gets

Attention Deficit Hyperactivity Disorder

(I include some books that are not specifically about children with ADHD but the antics and experiences of the children in them may strike a chord. Also I recommend all the *Ramona* books by Beverly Cleary, and all the *Soup* books by Robert Newton Peck.)

Alcott, L.M. *Little Men*. New York: The World Publishing Company.

Caudill, R. (1966) *Did You Carry the Flag Today, Charley?* New York: Holt, Rinehart & Winston.

Galvin, M. and Ferraro, S. (2001) *Otto Learns about his Medicine*. Washington, DC: Magination Press.

Gantos, J. (1998) *Joey Pigza Swallowed the Key*. New York: Harper Trophy.

Gantos, J. (2000) *Joey Pigza Loses Control*. New York: Farrar, Straus & Giroux.

Gehret, J. and Covert, S. (1996) *Eagle Eyes: A Child's View of Attention Deficit Disorder*. Fairport, NY: Verbal Images.

Nadeau, K.G., Littman, E. and Quinn, P. (1999) *Understanding Girls with ADHD*. Silver Spring, MD: Advantage Books.

Paulsen, G. (1993) *Harris and Me: A Summer Remembered*. San Diego, CA: Harcourt Brace.

Behavior Problems

Burch, R. (1967) *Queenie Peavy*. New York: Viking.

Cleary, B. (1999) *Otis Spofford*. New York: HarperCollins.

Gantos, J. (1980) *Rotten Ralph*. Boston, MA: Houghton Mifflin.

MacDonald, B. (1947) *Mrs. Piggle Wiggle* (and sequels). Philadelphia, PA: J.B. Lippincott.

Robinson, B. (1972) *The Best Christmas Pageant Ever*. New York: Harper & Row.

Sachar, L. (1987) *There's a Boy in the Girls' Bathroom*. New York: Alfred A. Knopf.

Sachar, L. (1991) *Dogs Don't Tell Jokes*. New York: Alfred A. Knopf.

Child Abuse (including physical, sexual, and verbal abuse)

Behm, B.J. and Anderson, E. (1999) *Tears of Joy*. Thiensville, WI: WayWord.

Crutcher, C. (1995) *Ironman*. New York: Greenwillow.

Gibbons, K. (1988) *Ellen Foster*. New York: Vintage.

Hoban, J. (1998) *Acting Normal.* New York: HarperCollins.

Magorian, M. (1982) *Goodnight, Mr. Tom.* New York: HarperCollins.

Quarles, H. (1998) *A Door Near Here.* New York: Delacorte.

Stanek, M. (1983) *Don't Hurt Me, Mama.* Niles, IL: Albert Whitman.

Voigt, C. (1994) *When She Hollers.* New York: Scholastic.

Developmental Delay

Keyes, D. (1995) *Flowers for Algernon.* New York: Harcourt.

McNey, M. and Fish, L. (1996) *Leslie's Story: A Book about a Girl with Mental Retardation.* Minneapolis, MN: Lerner.

Steinbeck, J. (1996) *Of Mice and Men.* New York: Chelsea House.

Movies
Bill
Bill: On his Own
Charley
Dominick and Eugene
Educating Peter
Forrest Gump
The Other Sister

Extraordinary Teachers

Braithwaite, E.R. (1959) *To Sir, with Love.* Englewood Cliffs, NJ: Prentice-Hall.

Conroy, P. (1972) *The Water is Wide.* Boston, MA: Houghton Mifflin.

Hayden, T.L. (1981) *Somebody Else's Kids.* New York: Putnam.

Johnson, L. (1995) *Dangerous Minds.* New York: St Martin's Press.

Kaufman, B. (1964) *Up the Down Staircase.* Englewood Cliffs, NJ: Prentice-Hall.

Kidder, T. (1989) *Among Schoolchildren.* Boston, MA: Houghton Mifflin.

Movies
Ciao, Professore!
Conrack
The Corn is Green
Dangerous Minds
Dead Poets' Society
Stand and Deliver
To Sir, with Love
Up the Down Staircase

Gifted and Talented Children

Brooks, B. (1986) *Midnight Hour Encores.* New York: Harper & Row.

Dahl, R. (1988) *Mathilda.* New York: Viking Kestrel.

Fitzhugh, L. (1967, 2000) *Harriet the Spy.* New York: Bantam Doubleday.

L'Engle, M. (1962) *A Wrinkle in Time.* New York: Ariel.

Paterson, K. (1985) *Come Sing, Jimmy Jo*. New York: Dutton.

Paterson, K. (1987) *Bridge to Terabithia*. New York: Harper Trophy.

Tevis, W.S. (1983) *The Queen's Gambit*. New York: Random House.

Movies

Finding Forrester

Good Will Hunting

Little Man Tate

October Sky

Searching for Bobby Fischer

Epilepsy

Moss, D.M. and Schwartz, C. (1989) *Lee, the Rabbit with Epilepsy*. Kensington, MD: Woodbine House.

Movie

The Basket

Siblings

Bach, A. (1980) *Waiting for Johnny Miracle*. New York: Harper & Row.

Gordon, M. (1992) *My Brother's a World-Class Pain: A Sibling's Guide to ADHD/Hyperactivity*. De Witt, NY: GSI (Gordon Systems, Inc.).

Meyer, D.J. (ed) (1997) *Views from Our Shoes: Growing Up with a Brother or Sister with Special Needs*. Bethesda, MD: Woodbine House.

Special Needs in General

Dwight, L. (1998) *We Can Do It!* New York: Star Bright Books.

Guralnick, M.J. (2000) *Interdisciplinary Clinical Assessment of Young Children with Developmental Disabilities*. Baltimore, MD: Paul H. Brookes.

Krementz, J. (1992) *How It Feels to Live with a Physical Disability*. New York: Simon & Schuster.

Nickel, R.E. and Desch. L.W. (eds) *2000) The Physician's Guide to Caring for Children with Disabilities and Chronic Conditions*. Baltimore, MD: Paul H. Brookes.

Rogers, F. (2000) *Extraordinary Friends: Let's Talk about It*. New York: Putnam.

Index

i16625481